Pegan Diet Cookbook

The best beginner's guide 100 Quick & Delicious Recipes to eat
Healthy food and Feel Great

ALICE FRANK

Table of Contents

INTRODUCTION 1

PEGAN DIET BENEFITS 2

BREAKFAST 5

1. Coconut and pistachio cream with blueberries 5

2. Cocoa and vanilla pancake 6

3. Coconut pancake 7

4. Coconut and cocoa pancake 8

5. Almond and berries pancake 9

6. Marble syrup and strawberries pancake 10

7. Cocoa and marble syrup pancake 11

8. Egg white and oat pancake 12

9. Egg white and vanilla pancake 13

10. Tofu and cinnamon pancake 14

11. Oat flour and banana pancake 15

12. Cocoa and banana pancake 16

13. Banana and almond pancake 17

14. Banana and pistachios pancake 18

15. Oat and cocoa pancake 19

16. Coconut and cocoa pancake 20

17. Oat and honey pancake 21

18. Oat and rice yogurt pancake 22

LUNCH RECIPES 23

19. Beef burger with cucumber, cherry tomatoes and onions. 23

20. Beef and zucchini 24

21. Beef and broccoli 25

22. Beef slices and cauliflower with coconut sauce 26

23. Beef with mushroom spicy sauce 27

24. Beef fillet with mushrooms and almonds 28

25. Flavoured chicken with baked cherry tomatoes 29

26. Chicken with tomatoes and avocado 30

27. Chicken stuffed with zucchini and tofu 31

28. Chicken in pistachio and almond crust 32

30. Pecans and tofu crusted turkey 34

31. Turkey and mushroom yogurt sauce 35

32. Turkey breast with vegetables 36

34. Salmon zucchini and mushrooms 38

35. Orange salmon and vegetables 39

36. Sesame seeds salmon 40

37. Salmon fillet and cinnamon raspberries 41

38. Lime cod and cherry tomatoes 42

40. Mint cod 44

41. Sea bass with lemon 45

42. Sea bass fillet with orange fennel 46

43. Almonds Mediterranean sea bass 47

SNACKS 48

44. Fruit salad with dried fruit 48

46. Fruit salad with strawberry sauce 50

47. Pineapple and strawberry fruit salad with mint 51

48. Detox smoothie 52

49. Smoothie bowl with kiwi and spinach 53

50. Peach smoothie 54

51. Ginger and melon smoothie 55

52. Peach and apricot smoothie 56

53. Watermelon and tofu skewers 57

54. Avocado and tomato tartare 58

55. Avocado and berries smoothie 59

56. Avocado and strawberry fruit salad 60

57. Pear and almond smoothie 61

60. Melon salad 64

61. Lime and ginger sorbet 65

62. Peach and carrot smoothie 66

63.   Vegan Golden Milk...67

64.   Smoothie bowl with apples, banana, and carrots 68

65.   Mint and cherries smoothie.. 69

DINNER RECIPES 70

66.   Beef burger with almonds, rocket salad and green beans . 70

67.   Beef with asparagus 71

68.   Orange beef and veggies...72

69.   Beef with cabbage...73

70.   Beef and fennels 74

71.   Beef and avocado..75

72.   Spicy chicken and broccoli...76

73.   Chicken broccoli roulade...77

74.   Chicken and bell peppers.. 78

75.   Avocado orange chicken 80

76.   Mushroom chicken thighs 81

77.   Almond chicken with olives and mushrooms 83

78.   Tofu turkey and veggies 84

79.   Turkey with tomatoes and bell peppers 85

80.   Turkey and vegetable salad... 87

81.   Pecans and tofu crusted salmon..88

82.   Almond crusted salmon 89

83.   Salmon burger 90

84.   Salmon and avocado salad...91

85.   Orange smoked salmon and mushrooms salad................. 92

86.   Cod fillet and veggies 93

87.   Flavoured herbs cod 94

88.   Hazelnut crusted cod 95

89.   Sea bass and cherry tomatoes 96

90.   Kiwi salad 97

91.   Corn soup..98

92.   Potato soup with Saffron 99

93. Brown rice with tomato 100

94. Turmeric potatoes 101

95. Sweet and sour fennel 102

96. Avocado and cucumber tartare 103

97. Salad of cucumbers, radishes, rocket and olives...........104

98. Orange seitan steaks..105

99. Grilled tofu and beetroot skewers...............................106

100. Spicy grilled zucchini 107

101. Zucchini, peppers and mushrooms in a pan..................108

102. Pumpkin in a pan with onions....................................109

103. Green beans, potatoes and zucchini 110

104. Peppers and green beans 111

105. Brown rice with vegetables and olives........................112

106. Seitan with mango..113

107. Potato and caper salad..114

INTRODUCTION

Going on a diet is never easy. There are various obstacles that we should face and these obstacles, most of the time, make our job really harder. Furthermore, we need a strong will that allows us to follow a dietary diet consistently. In fact, we must always find the right determination and motivation that push us to move forward and to pursue our main goal, which is weight loss. And when it always comes to proposing a diet, it is even more difficult to find a meal plan that can reflect everyone's needs and preferences. Because there are those who prefer certain foods or those who, for a purely personal choice, decide not to eat certain foods. We are talking about those who, for their own conscience, have scruples in eating meat or fish, or those who do not want to eat anything that is of animal origin. We are talking about those who have embraced the vegan philosophy by placing it as a style not only for food but also for whole life. However, it is known that some diets, especially the most successful ones, often involve the sacrifice of a macronutrient, such as carbohydrates, to allow greater weight loss. It is therefore often high-protein diets with a large amount of proteins of animal origin. Having said that, one important question could be if there is a combination of these different factors and different needs. To help this question, the Pegan diet was devised. Pegan is a diet that offers an unusual combination of a Paleo diet and a Vegan diet. If you look closely at the word itself, you understand that it is the fusion of the Paleo and Vegan diets. We are talking about two dietary protocols that have been very successful in recent years and attracted many followers. This is because they not only work at the weight loss level but also because of the health benefits that both of these diets bring us. The main objective of this text is to explain what the Pegan diet is, and how this perfect combination of two diets works if they are very different from each other, both philosophically and practically. No less important will be the goal of understanding this diet in order to have a good general nutritional education. You will understand how nutritional education can bring benefits not only on a physical and metabolic level, but also in mentally. Speaking specifically about the division of the book in the first part of the text, you will find all the basic explanations: features and origins of the Pegan diet, its benefits and the philosophy behind this sensational dietary protocol. As, for the benefits, there will be a part that will discuss the benefits of the Pegan diet for people with more or less severe diseases such as those who are hypertensive or have diabetes. In the second

1

part you will find a section dedicated to pregnant women where you will be advised more specifically what to add or decrease. In addition to pregnant women there will be a chapter dedicated to sportsmen: in this part, there will be some tricks for those who play sports but we will also try to make you understand a fundamental concept. This fundamental concept is linked to the fact that, for the success of any diet, it is always important to accompany it with adequate physical activity. There will then be a third part where you will find practical advice on how to create your perfect meal plan. There will also be a part dedicated to the shopping list, so on, which foods are allowed, and which ones are forbidden. You will also find indications on how to apply the subsequent recipes to the meal plan. Finally, the fourth and last part will be completely dedicated to recipes: in fact, you will find 300 easy-to-make recipes aimed especially at those who have little time and work. At the end of the reading, you will be perfectly aware of how this diet works, the tools to make it, what to eat and not to eat and the food plans and recipes to follow

PEGAN DIET BENEFITS

What are Pegan diet main benefits? After examining the characteristics, origins and philosophy behind the Pegan diet, it is time to show you all the benefits you can take from this diet. In this first paragraph we will only deal with the general benefits that this diet can bring, while in the second we will talk about the specific benefits for certain types of diseases. However, the general benefits of this diet are: • First, it is a healthy food protocol. As we have already said, the Pegan diet reflects a healthy and balanced diet that meets all nutritional needs. Although it is a regime that is always against carbohydrates in favour of proteins and fats, thanks to the contribution of vegetables, it provides vitamins and minerals that are not present in other low-carb diets. This diet does not exclude any essential ingredient for the body. On the contrary, it provides in a balanced way all the nutrients it needs to have energy and function at its best. • It is a diet that benefits health in general, as it is a regime designed for the general well-being of our body: from improving the condition of the stomach and liver to that of our mind. You will not only notice an improvement in your digestive condition or your better skin but also an improvement in mental performance. You will realize that you are much more focused, and succeed better, for example if you do a job that requires more mental effort. In addition,

2

thanks to the increased intake of fruit and vegetables, there is an increase in the consumption of fibre with a positive impact on heart health and the reduction of diseases (especially in the colon). • It is a long-term diet: linked to the above, being a balanced diet that positively affects general health it could become a protocol (unlike other low carb diets such as Keto which must be followed only for a short period to avoid damage in the body) to be followed for a long time. It is not for nothing that Pegan is also defined as the 365 diet: a diet that can be followed throughout the year. This is because, as we have already seen, it is based on an annual formula with a balance of proteins, vegetables, good fats and fibres, decreasing the imbalance in favor of carbohydrates as you go along. • It is suitable for everyone. The Pegan diet, having been studied with the purpose of responding to a multitude of needs, turns out to be a diet that can be used by everyone. • It is a diet that follows a pattern but that can be customized: we now know that Pegan is also based on a quick formula for personalizing meals: the formula of 5-4-3-2-1, are a series of numbers, a way to balance proteins, carbohydrates and vegetables, fats and fibres.
• It still allows short-term results: even if it is a style, that can be adopted and projected over the long term, the Pegan diet allows for weight loss results and improvement of health in general right away. It is still a low-carb protocol that aims at rapid weight loss. • Improves the conditions of the metabolism: thanks to the fact that it is a diet that aims at food re-education, it will certainly affect the performance of your metabolism. Choosing unprocessed, low-glycaemic foods with the right amount of nutrients will also fix a malfunctioning metabolism. Combined with sport, it will become the ideal ally for long-term results also with regard to our "metabolic machine". • Reduces stress eating: managing to keep blood sugar under control by not increasing the level of sugar in the blood, this diet allows you to drastically reduce the dependence on sugars themselves. Moreover, it is well known, that this addiction is the main cause of stress eating. • It completely renews not only our eating style but also our lifestyle: being a regime that aims at food re-education that is to make us understand what is healthier to eat for us, this diet can only become a real style of life. The idea behind the Pegan diet is to eliminate processed and industrial foods from your life as well as sugars and starches in favour of plant foods, foods rich in proteins and healthy fats. In reality, foods of animal origin are not completely excluded; in fact, they can be consumed as long as they

3

come from organic and sustainable farms. It is therefore a matter of choosing the ingredients selectively and personally cooking our meals. This new way of thinking about the foods we eat will inevitably affect our habits and lifestyle. • The Pegan diet is a low environmental impact diet: this is because it proposes to choose as much local and organic food as possible in order to avoid chemicals, additives and pesticides. All this also has a lower impact on the health of the environment around us. These that we have listed are all the possible benefits in general that the Pegan diet can bring. In the next chapter, we will describe and show you all the advantages that specifically concern diabetes and cardiovascular diseases (such as hypertension).

BREAKFAST

1. Coconut and pistachio cream with blueberries

PREPARATION TIME: 5 minutes REST TIME: 30 minutes
CALORIES: 380

INGREDIENTS FOR 2 SERVINGS

200 ml of coconut milk with no added sugar 40 grams of
blueberries 4 tablespoons of chia seeds 2 tablespoons of
coconut flour 2 tablespoons of pistachio flour (or finely
chopped pistachios) 1 pinch of vanilla powder

DIRECTIONS

First, mix the coconut milk, chia seeds, coconut flour, pistachio
flour and vanilla powder in a bowl. Beat the ingredients until
the mixture has completely thickened. Pour the mixture equally
into two bowls. Let it rest for half an hour in the fridge. After
this time, take your coconut and pistachio creams and sprinkle
them with other chia seeds. In the meantime, wash the
blueberries. Serve your cream accompanied by blueberries.

2. Cocoa and vanilla pancake

PREPARATION TIME: 10 minutes COOKING TIME: 5 minutes CALORIES: 150

INGREDIENTS FOR 2 SERVINGS

50 grams of almond flour 1 egg 10 grams sugar free cocoa powder 4 drops of sweetener (such us Stevia) 30 ml sugar-free almond milk 1 ml of vanilla extract 1 pinch of baking soda Coconut oil to taste

DIRECTIONS

First, separate the yolk from the egg white and transfer them into two different bowls. 2   Add the sweetener drops to the yolk and beat with a whisk. 3   Add the almond milk and beat again. 4   Then add the almond flour, vanilla extract, baking soda and sifted bitter cocoa. 5   Mix until all the ingredients will be smooth. 6   Then whip the egg whites until stiff and gently incorporate them into the rest of the dough. 7   Heat a non-stick pan and grease it lightly with coconut oil. 8   Pour a spoonful of dough for each pancake and wait about a minute. 9 After that time, you can turn them over and continue cooking on the other side. 10   Continue to cook all the pancakes like this. 11   Serve the pancakes still hot.

3. Coconut pancake

PREPARATION TIME: 10 minutes COOKING TIME: 5 minutes CALORIES: 170

INGREDIENTS FOR 2 SERVINGS

30 grams of almond flour 20 grams of coconut flour 1 big egg drops of sweetener (such us Stevia) 30 ml of sugar-free coconut milk 1 pinch of baking soda 1 pinch of cinnamon 1 teaspoon of Coconut oil

DIRECTIONS

First, separate the yolk from the egg white and transfer them into two different bowls. 2   Add the sweetener drops to the yolk and beat with a whisk. 3   Add the coconut milk and beat again. 4   Then add the almond flour, coconut flour, cinnamon and baking soda. 5   Mix until all the ingredients will be smooth. 6   Heat a non-stick pan and grease it lightly with coconut oil. 7   Pour a spoonful of dough for each pancake and wait about a minute. 8   As soon as the first bubbles form, you can turn them over and continue cooking on the other side. 9   Continue to cook all the pancakes like this. 10   Serve the pancakes still hot with coconut flour pour over.

4. Coconut and cocoa pancake

PREPARATION TIME: 10 minutes COOKING TIME: 5 minutes CALORIES: 190

INGREDIENTS FOR 2 SERVINGS

25 grams of almond flour 20 grams of coconut flour grams of sugar free cocoa powder 1 big egg 4 drops of sweetener (such us Stevia) 30 ml of sugar-free coconut milk 1 pinch of baking soda Olive oil to taste

DIRECTIONS

First, separate the yolk from the egg white and transfer them into two different bowls. 2   Add the sweetener drops to the yolk and beat with a whisk. 3   Add the coconut milk and beat again. 4   Then add the almond flour, coconut flour, cocoa powder and baking soda. 5   Mix until all the ingredients will be smooth. 6   Heat a non-stick pan and grease it lightly. 7 Pour a spoonful of dough for each pancake and wait about a minute. 8   As soon as the first bubbles form, you can turn them over and continue cooking on the other side. 9 Continue to cook all the pancakes like this. 10   Serve the pancakes still hot with coconut flour pour over.

5. Almond and berries pancake

PREPARATION TIME: 10 minutes COOKING TIME: 5 minutes
CALORIES: 220

INGREDIENTS FOR 2 SERVINGS

50 grams of almond flour 1 egg 6 drops of sweetener 30 ml of
sugar-free almond milk 1 pinch of baking soda 1 pinch of
nutmeg 50 grams of berries 30 grams of chopped almonds
olive oil to taste

DIRECTIONS

Start dividing the yolk from the egg white and transfer them to
two different bowls. 2   Add the sweetener drops to the yolk
and beat with a whisk. 3   Also, add the almond milk and
continue beating. 4   Then add the almond flour, baking soda
and nutmeg. 5   Stir until you have a smooth mixture.
6   Then whip the egg whites until stiff and gently incorporate
them into the rest of the dough. 7   Heat a non-stick pan and
grease it lightly. 8   Pour a spoonful of dough for each
pancake and wait about a minute. 9   As soon as the first
bubbles form, you can turn them over and continue cooking on
the other side. 10   Continue to cook all the pancakes like this.
11   Meanwhile peel and chop almonds. 12   Serve pancake
turrets with berries and chopped almonds.

6. Marble syrup and strawberries pancake

PREPARATION TIME: 10 minutes COOKING TIME: 5 minutes CALORIES: 220

INGREDIENTS FOR 2 SERVINGS

25 grams of almond flour 15 grams of oat flour 1 small egg 4 drops of sweetener 30 ml of sugar-free soymilk 1 pinch of baking soda 1 pinch nutmeg 50 grams of strawberries 2 teaspoons of low carb sugar free marble syrup olive oil to taste

DIRECTIONS

Start dividing the yolk from the egg white and transfer them to two different bowls. 2.   Add the sweetener drops to the yolk and beat with a whisk. 3.   Also, add the soymilk and keep on melting. 4.   Then add the all powder ingredients (almond flour, oat flour, baking soda and nutmeg). 5.   Smooth all ingredients. 6.   Then whip the egg whites until stiff and gently incorporate them into the rest of the dough. 7.   Heat a non-stick pan and grease it lightly. 8.   Pour a spoonful of dough for each pancake and wait about a minute. 9.   As soon as the first bubbles form, you can turn them over and continue cooking on the other side. 10. Continue to cook all the pancakes like this. 11. Meanwhile wash strawberries, then halve. 12. Serve pancake with strawberries and marble syrup pour over.

7. Cocoa and marble syrup pancake

PREPARATION TIME: 10 minutes COOKING TIME: 5 minutes
CALORIES: 210

INGREDIENTS FOR 2 SERVINGS

50 grams of almond flour grams of sugar free cocoa powder 1
big egg 4 drops of sweetener (such us Stevia) 35 ml of sugar-
free coconut milk 1 pinch of baking soda 1 tsp low carb sugar
free marble syrup Olive oil to taste

DIRECTIONS

Start placing the egg white into a large bowl. Add the sweetener
drops and beat with a whisk. Add the coconut milk and beat
again. Then add the almond flour, cocoa powder and baking
soda. Mix until all the ingredients will be smooth. Heat a non-
stick pan and grease it lightly. Pour a spoonful of dough for
each pancake and wait about a minute. After 1 minute, you can
turn them over and continue cooking on the other side.
Continue to cook all the pancakes like this. Serve the pancakes
with a topping off marble syrup.

8. Egg white and oat pancake

PREPARATION TIME: 10 minutes COOKING TIME: 5 minutes CALORIES: 190

INGREDIENTS FOR 2 SERVINGS

50 grams of oat flour 2 eggs white 6 drops of sweetener 30 ml of sugar-free coconut milk A pinch of baking soda Olive oil to taste

DIRECTIONS

Start placing the eggs white into a large bowl. Add the sweetener drops and beat with a whisk. Add the coconut milk and beat again. Then add the oat flour and baking soda. Mix until all the ingredients will be smooth. Heat a non-stick pan and grease it lightly. Pour a spoonful of dough for each pancake and wait about a minute. As soon as the first bubbles form, you can turn them over and continue cooking on the other side. Continue to cook all the pancakes like this. Serve still hot.

9. Egg white and vanilla pancake

PREPARATION TIME: 10 minutes COOKING TIME: 5 minutes
CALORIES: 190

INGREDIENTS FOR 2 SERVINGS

50 grams of almond flour 2 eggs white 6 drops of sweetener
30 ml of sugar-free soymilk 5 ml of vanilla extract A pinch of
baking soda Olive oil to taste

DIRECTIONS

Start placing the eggs white into a large bowl. Add the
sweetener drops and beat with a whisk. Add the soymilk,
vanilla extract and beat again. Then add the almond flour and
baking soda. Mix until all the ingredients will be smooth. Heat
a non-stick pan and grease it lightly. Pour a spoonful of dough
for each pancake and wait about a minute. As soon as the first
bubbles form, you can turn them over and continue cooking on
the other side. Continue to cook all the pancakes like this.
Serve still hot.

10.   Tofu and cinnamon pancake

PREPARATION TIME: 10 minutes COOKING TIME: 5 minutes CALORIES: 270

INGREDIENTS FOR 2 SERVINGS

2 eggs 100 grams of tofu, cubed ml of water 60 grams of almond flour 2 grams of baking powder 5 ml of vanilla extract ½ teaspoon of cinnamon 1/2 teaspoon stevia sweetener 2 tablespoons of coconut oil

DIRECTIONS

Add all ingredients to a blender. 2   Start with eggs and water and tofu cheese so you do not have anything is stuck at bottom. 3   Blend until smooth, scraping down the sides if needed. 4 Let batter sit for 2 minutes. 5   Heat a non-stick skillet to medium heat. 6   For each pancake, pour 2 tablespoons of coconut oil onto skillet. 7   Once you start to see little bubbles form, flip and continue to cook until pancake is browned on each side. 8   Continue until you have used all pancake batter. 9   Serve pancakes hot.

11. Oat flour and banana pancake

PREPARATION TIME: 10 minutes COOKING TIME: 5 minutes
CALORIES: 180

INGREDIENTS FOR 2 SERVINGS

70 grams of oat flour ½ banana 1 teaspoon of baking soda 8
drops of sweetener (such us Stevia) 15 ml of rice milk 1 pinch if
cinnamon seed oil to taste

DIRECTIONS

First, peel and mash the half banana until you get a mush. Add
the sweetener drops to the mix and beat with a whisk. Add the
rice milk and beat again. Then add the oat flour, baking soda
and cinnamon. Mix until all the ingredients will be smooth.
Then whip the egg whites until stiff and gently incorporate them
into the rest of the dough. Heat a non-stick pan and grease it
lightly. Pour a spoonful of dough for each pancake and wait
about a minute. As soon as the first bubbles form, you can turn
them over and continue cooking on the other side. Continue to
cook all the pancakes like this. Serve the pancakes still hot.

12. Cocoa and banana pancake

PREPARATION TIME: 10 minutes COOKING TIME: 5 minutes CALORIES: 180

INGREDIENTS FOR 2 SERVINGS

50 grams of oat flour 30 grams of sugar free cocoa powder Banana 1 teaspoon of baking soda 4 drops of sweetener (such us Stevia) 15 ml of soymilk 1 pinch if cinnamon Vegetal oil to taste

DIRECTIONS

First, peel and mash the banana until you get a mush. Add the sweetener drops to the mix and beat with a whisk. Add the soymilk and beat again. Then add the oat flour, baking soda and cinnamon. Mix until all the ingredients will be smooth. Then whip the egg whites until stiff and gently incorporate them into the rest of the dough. Heat a non-stick pan and grease it lightly. Pour a spoonful of dough for each pancake and wait about a minute. As soon as the first bubbles form, you can turn them over and continue cooking on the other side. Continue to cook all the pancakes like this. Serve the pancakes still hot.

13. Banana and almond pancake

PREPARATION TIME: 10 minutes COOKING TIME: 5 minutes CALORIES: 200

INGREDIENTS FOR 2 SERVINGS

60 grams of almond flour ½ banana 20 ml of almond milk 5 ml of lemon juice 2 grams of baking soda 2 teaspoons of low carb marble syrup olive oil to taste 20 grams of chopped almonds (to serve)

DIRECTIONS

Start by peeling and slicing half banana. Then put banana slices in a mix and blend until obtain a thick cream. Add the lemon juice to the banana cream and beat with a whisk. Add the almond milk and beat again. Then add the almond flour and baking soda. Mix until all the ingredients will be smooth. Then whip the egg whites until stiff and gently incorporate them into the rest of the dough. Heat a non-stick pan and grease it lightly. Pour a spoonful of dough for each pancake and wait about a minute. As soon as the first bubbles form, you can turn them over and continue cooking on the other side. Continue to cook all the pancakes like this. Meanwhile, chop almonds. Serve the pancakes still hot with a topping of marble syrup and chopped almonds.

14. Banana and pistachios pancake

PREPARATION TIME: 10 minutes COOKING TIME: 5 minutes CALORIES: 210

INGREDIENTS FOR 2 SERVINGS

50 grams of almond flour 10 grams of oat flour 1 teaspoon of pistachio flour (or finely chopped pistachios) ½ banana 40 ml of soymilk 5 ml of orange juice 2 grams of baking soda 2 teaspoons of low carb marble syrup olive oil to taste 20 grams of chopped pistachios (to serve)

DIRECTIONS Start by peeling and slicing half banana. Then put banana slices in a mix and blend until obtain a thick cream. Add the orange juice to the banana cream and beat with a whisk. Add the soymilk and beat again. Then add the almond, oat and pistachios flour and baking soda. If you don't' have pistachios flour, you can chop finely 30 grams of pistachios, so you will have all of them for the whole recipe. Mix until all the ingredients will be smooth. Then whip the egg whites until stiff and gently incorporate them into the rest of the dough. Heat a non-stick pan and grease it lightly. Pour a spoonful of dough for each pancake and wait about a minute. As soon as the first bubbles form, you can turn them over and continue cooking on the other side. Continue to cook all the pancakes like this.

Serve the pancakes still hot with a topping of marble syrup and chopped pistachios.

15. Oat and cocoa pancake

PREPARATION TIME: 10 minutes COOKING TIME: 5 minutes CALORIES: 180

INGREDIENTS FOR 2 SERVINGS

60 grams of oat flour 100 ml of soy yogurt 20 ml of soymilk 1 teaspoon of sugar free cocoa powder 1 pinch of baking soda ½ teaspoon of vanilla extract Coconut oil to taste

DIRECTIONS

First, put the soy yogurt in a large bowl. Add the vanilla extract and beat with a whisk. Add the soymilk too and beat again. Then add the oat flour, baking soda and sifted bitter cocoa. Mix until all the ingredients will be smooth. Then whip the egg whites until stiff and gently incorporate them into the rest of the dough. Heat a non-stick pan and grease it lightly. Pour a spoonful of dough for each pancake and wait about a minute. As soon as the first bubbles form, you can turn them over and continue cooking on the other side. Continue to cook all the pancakes like this. Serve pancakes still hot.

16. Coconut and cocoa pancake

PREPARATION TIME: 10 minutes COOKING TIME: 5 minutes CALORIES: 220

INGREDIENTS FOR 2 SERVINGS

40 grams of oat flour 30 grams of coconut flour 100 ml of coconut milk 1 teaspoon of soymilk 10 grams of sugar free cocoa powder 1 pinch of baking soda 1 pinch of cinnamon Coconut oil to taste

DIRECTIONS

First, put the coconut milk in a large bowl. Add the cinnamon and beat with a whisk. Add the soymilk too and beat again. Then add the oat flour, coconut flour, baking soda and sifted bitter cocoa. Then whip the egg whites until stiff and gently incorporate them into the rest of the dough. Heat a non-stick pan and grease it lightly with coconut oil. Pour a spoonful of dough for each pancake and wait about a minute. As soon as the first bubbles form, you can turn them over and continue cooking on the other side. Continue to cook all the pancakes like this. Serve pancakes still hot.

17. Oat and honey pancake

PREPARATION TIME: 10 minutes COOKING TIME: 5 minutes
CALORIES: 190

INGREDIENTS FOR 2 SERVINGS

60 grams of oat flour 10 ml of (100% biological) honey 50 ml of
soy yogurt 1 pinch of vanilla powder 2 drops of sweeteners
such stevia 20 ml of sugar-free soymilk 1 pinch of baking soda
Olive oil to taste

DIRECTIONS

First, put the soy yogurt in a large bowl and beat with a whisk.
Add the soymilk too and honey, then beat again. Then add the
oat flour, stevia, baking soda and vanilla powder. Mix until all
the ingredients will be smooth. Then whip the egg whites until
stiff and gently incorporate them into the rest of the dough.
Heat a non-stick pan and grease it lightly. Pour a spoonful of
dough for each pancake and wait about a minute. As soon as
the first bubbles form, you can turn them over and continue
cooking on the other side. Continue to cook all the pancakes
like this. Serve still hot.

18.Oat and rice yogurt pancake

PREPARATION TIME: 10 minutes COOKING TIME: 5 minutes CALORIES: 190

INGREDIENTS FOR 2 SERVINGS

60 grams of oat flour 50 ml of vegan rice yogurt 1 pinch of cinnamon ½ teaspoon of powder stevia 20 ml of sugar-free rice milk 1 pinch of baking soda Coconut oil to taste

DIRECTIONS

First, put the rice yogurt in a large bowl and beat with a whisk. Add the rice milk too and beat again. Then add the oat flour, stevia, baking soda and cinnamon. Mix until all the ingredients will be smooth. Then whip the egg whites until stiff and gently incorporate them into the rest of the dough. Heat a non-stick pan and grease it lightly with coconut oil. Pour a spoonful of dough for each pancake and wait about a minute. As soon as the first bubbles form, you can turn them over and continue cooking on the other side. Continue to cook all the pancakes like this. Serve still hot

LUNCH RECIPES

19. Beef burger with cucumber, cherry tomatoes and onions.

PREPARATION TIME: 20 minutes COOKING TIME: 6 minutes
CALORIES: 353

INGREDIENTS FOR 2 SERVINGS

2 beef burgers of 150 grams each 50 grams of cherry tomatoes
50 grams of rocket Half a red onion 1 small cucumber 1 clove
of garlic 100 gr of non-diary yogurt Olive oil to taste Salt and
pepper to taste

DIRECTIONS

Wash and dry the cucumber and then divide it in two
horizontally. Cut one-half into cubes and the other into slices.
Peel the garlic clove, wash it, and chop it. Put the yogurt, garlic,
diced cucumber, salt, and pepper in a bowl and mix well. Put
the bowl in the fridge until the rest of the ingredients are ready.
Peel the onion, wash it and then cut it into thin slices. Wash
and pat the rocket. Wash the cherry tomatoes and then cut
them into 4 parts. Now take the burgers and brush them with a
little olive oil. Heat up a grill and then put the hamburger to
grill for 3 minutes per side. Put the burgers on 2 serving plates.

Garnish with the vegetables, season with oil, salt and pepper and then sprinkle everything with the yogurt sauce and serve.

20.   Beef and zucchini

PREPARATION TIME: 10 minutes COOKING TIME: 20 minutes CALORIES: 410

INGREDIENTS FOR 2 SERVINGs

2 beef fillets (200 grams about for each) 3 tablespoons of olive oil ½ lime 1 zucchini 40 ml of water 1 pinch of Italian seasoning 1/2 shallot 3 grams of chives Salt and pepper to taste 1 pinch of smoked paprika 10 grams of chopped parsley

DIRECTIONS Peel the zucchini, then wash and dry it. Cut it into little cubes. Peel and wash the shallot too. Dry it and then chop it. Take a non-stick pan and heat the oil. When it is hot, add the zucchini and brown it for 4 minutes, seasoning with salt and Italian seasoning. Add water and let cook for other 10 minutes or until water will be absorbed. Let zucchini drain. Wash and dry the fillet and then cut it into small pieces. Wash and dry the lime, grate the peel and set it aside and then squeeze the pulp and strain the juice into a bowl. Put the meat, salt, pepper, chives, olive oil, paprika, and parsley in the bowl with the lime juice. Stir gently to mix everything. Let sauté the beef filet with the sauce for few minutes in a pan. When it will be done, serve the meat in the centre of the plate. Add the zucchini cubes and serve.

21. Beef and broccoli

PREPARATION TIME: 10 minutes COOKING TIME: 20 minutes CALORIES: 450

INGREDIENTS FOR 2 SERVINGS

400 grams of Beef fillet 12 broccoli tops 1sprigs of thyme
½ lemon juice 10 ml of olive oil Salt and pepper to taste

DIRECTIONS

Wash and dry broccoli tops, then cut them into many pieces. Remove any excess fat from the beef, then wash and dry it. Wash and dry thyme sprigs. Put the olive oil, lemon, salt and pepper in a bowl and mix with a fork until you get a homogeneous emulsion. Take one sheet of aluminium foil and place the beef. Add the broccoli, thyme and then wet everything with the oil and lemon emulsion. Close the foil making sure to seal it well. Put in the oven and cook at 180°c for 15/20 minutes. When it is ready, remove the thyme, serve beef fillet with the broccoli, and sprinkled with the marinating liquid.

22.   Beef slices and cauliflower with coconut sauce

PREPARATION TIME: 15 minutes COOKING TIME: 10 minutes CALORIES: 480

INGREDIENTS FOR 2 SERVINGS

350 grams of beef fillet sliced 1/4 inch thick 200 grams of cauliflower florets 20 ml of olive oil 10 grams of minced garlic 1 teaspoon of ginger powder For the sauce: 100 ml of water 20 ml of coconut milk 10 ml of sesame oil 10 ml of beef stock

DIRECTIONS First, peel garlic clove and mince it. Wash and cut cauliflower into florets and set aside. Wash and dry beef fillet too. Slice beef into 1/4 inch slices. Measure ingredients for sauce into a small bowl. Bring everything to the stove. Heat skillet or wok over medium-high heat. When hot, add half of the olive oil and swirl to coat the pan. When the oil shimmers, add the beef, cooking for 30 seconds on the first side before turning over to continue cooking. Remove to a plate or bowl and keep warm. Add the remaining olive oil to the pan with the garlic and ginger. Stir until fragrant. Then add the sauce and cauliflower giving it a quick stir. Cover to steam until the cauliflower is crisp tender. Remove. Add any accumulated meat juices to the pan and reduce sauce to a few tablespoons. Add the beef and cauliflower back to the pan to warm through. Season with salt and pepper to taste and serve.

23. Beef with mushroom spicy sauce

PREPARATION TIME: 15 minutes COOKING TIME: 20 minutes CALORIES: 380

INGREDIENTS FOR 2 SERVINGS

350 grams of beef fillet 200 grams of mushrooms 50 ml of vegetal cooking cream 1 garlic clove 1 tablespoon olive oil 1 tsp mix of spices Salt to taste.

DIRECTIONS

Peel and wash the garlic. Remove the earthy part of the mushrooms, wash them under running water, dry them and then cut them into slices. Clean the beef fillet. Remove excess fat and then cut into two slices. Wash it and dry it. Heat the olive oil in a pan. As soon as it is hot, brown the garlic and then remove it. Place the beef slices and brown them on both sides until they are well cooked. Season with salt, pepper and mix of spices. Remove the beef and keep it warm. Now add the mushrooms to the pan where you cooked the beef before. Brown them for 10 minutes and then add the cream. Stir to mix well, Let the sauce reduce and then season with salt and pepper. Add the beef fillet, let it flavour and then turn off the heat. Serve the fillet sprinkled with the mushroom sauce.

24. Beef fillet with mushrooms and almonds

PREPARATION TIME: 10 minutes COOKING TIME: 20 minutes CALORIES: 430

INGREDIENTS FOR 2 SERVINGS 2 beef fillets (200 grams for each) 200 grams of mushrooms 10 ml of olive oil 1 garlic clove (minced) Salt and pepper to taste. 5 grams of chopped parsley 30 grams if chopped almonds

DIRECTIONSStart by cleaning the mushrooms. Remove the earthy part, wash them well under running water, dry them and then cut them into thin slices. Clean the beef filet. Remove the excess fat or if still present the calloused part and then wash it under running water and dry it with absorbent paper. Peel and wash the garlic, then mince it. Heat the oil in a pan. As soon as it is hot enough, fry the garlic. As soon as the garlic has taken on a golden colour, put the beef in the pan. Cook the fillet for 3 minutes on both sides, making sure to seal the meat well. Season with salt and pepper. After the cooking time, put the fillet to rest so that it remains warm anyway. In the same pan where you browned the fillets, now cook the mushrooms. Cook them for 6 minutes, stirring occasionally, then add the salt and pepper and cook for another 10 minutes. Meanwhile, wash, dry and finely chop the parsley. Finely chop the almonds too. When the mushrooms are ready, take two serving plates, place one fillet per plate, surround with the mushrooms and sprinkle them with the mushroom sauce. Finish garnishing with the chopped parsley and the chopped almonds and serve.

25. Flavoured chicken with baked cherry tomatoes

PREPARATION TIME: 20 minutes+ 30 minutes to marinate
COOKING TIME: 20 minutes CALORIES: 337

INGREDIENTS FOR 2 SERVINGS 300 grams of chicken breast 200 grams of cherry tomatoes 1 clove of garlic 1 sprig of rosemary 1 bay leaf Half a lemon A teaspoon of dried oregano Salt and pepper to taste Olive oil to taste

DIRECTIONS Wash and dry the chicken breast, remove fat and bones, and then divide it in half. Wash and dry thyme, rosemary, and bay leaves. Wash and dry the cherry tomatoes and leave them whole and then chop them. Peel the garlic and chop it. Wash the lemon, remove the zest, and cut it into slices. Put the lemon juice, two tablespoons of olive oil, salt, pepper and the aromatic herbs in a bowl and mix. Add the chicken and let it marinate for 30 minutes. Take a baking sheet and brush it with olive oil. Put the chicken inside and then the cherry tomatoes. Sprinkle everything with the chicken marinade and the lemon strips and then cook in the oven at 200 ° C for 20 minutes. As soon as it is cooked, take it out of the oven, put the chicken and the cherry tomatoes on the plate, sprinkle with the cooking juices and serve.

26.   Chicken with tomatoes and avocado

PREPARATION TIME: 15 minutes + 20 minutes of marinating in the fridge COOKING TIME: 10 minutes CALORIES: 420

INGREDIENTS FOR 2 SERVINGS

400 grams of chicken breast, sliced. 1 little orange 1 shallot 20 cherry tomatoes 1 avocado 1 teaspoon of dried oregano Salt and pepper to taste. 10 ml of coconut oil

DIRECTIONS

Wash and dry chicken breast then cut it into slices. Transfer the chicken to a large pan and season with coconut oil, salt and pepper. Squeeze the orange and strain the juice. Then sprinkle the chicken slices. Add the aromatic herbs too and mix the slices to flavour them well. Cover with transparent paper and put them in the fridge for 20 minutes to marinate. Wash and dry the cherry tomatoes and then cut them into cubes. Peel the shallot, wash it and chop it. Peel the avocado, remove the stone, wash it, dry it and then cut it into cubes. Put the tomatoes, avocado, and shallot in a bowl, season with oil, salt and pepper and mix. After 20 minutes, remove the chicken from the fridge. Heat a grill, which should be hot, and cook the slices for 3 minutes per side. The chicken should be well cooked and have grill streaks on the surface. Transfer the chicken to serving plates and garnish with the avocado and cherry tomato mixture.

27.　Chicken stuffed with zucchini and tofu

PREPARATION TIME: 15 minutes COOKING TIME: 25 minutes CALORIES: 380

INGREDIENTS FOR 2 SERVINGS

4 chicken breast slices 1 zucchini 2 sage leaves 40 grams of tofu (cubed) 20 ml of olive oil Salt and cayenne pepper to taste.

DIRECTIONS

Start with the zucchini. Wash it, dry it and then cut it into thin slices. Put a pot with a little salted water, and when it comes to a boil, boil the zucchini slices for 3 minutes. Drain and put them to cool. Switch to the chicken slices, beating them with a meat tenderizer to thin them, washing and dry them. Wash and dry the sage too. Meanwhile cut tofu into little cubes. Put the zucchini first and then tofu on each slice. Roll the meat on itself and stop the roll with a toothpick. Heat the olive oil in a non-stick pan. As soon as it is hot, add the sage leaves and then the rolls. Cook them until the outside of the slices are golden brown and the meat well cooked. Season with salt and cayenne pepper and turn off the heat. Serve stuffed chicken still hot.

28.   Chicken in pistachio and almond crust

PREPARATION TIME: 10minutes COOKING TIME: 20 minutes CALORIES: 420

INGREDIENTS FOR 2 SERVINGS

350 grams of chicken breast 60 grams of chopped pistachios 20 grams of chopped almonds The juice of an orange orange zest 5 grams of chopped rosemary 20 ml of olive oil Salt and pepper to taste

DIRECTIONS Start with cleaning the chicken breast. Wash it, dry it and remove any bone or excess fat. Cut chicken breast in 2 parts. Wash the orange peel and then cut them into thin slices. Put together the pistachios, almonds and rosemary on a plate. Stir and combine them well. Bread chicken breasts with the dried fruit breading pressing well with your fingertips to make it adhere evenly. Heat the olive oil in a pan. Brown chicken breasts, cooking it for at least 10 minutes on each side. Season with salt and pepper, then remove the fillets from the heat and keep them warm. In the same pan, prepare the accompanying sauce. Add the orange juice, a tablespoon of water, a drizzle of olive oil, salt and pepper and let it reduce by half, stirring so that the sauce does not burn. Take two serving plates, put the orange sauce on the bottom of the plate, lay the chicken on top and serve surrounded with orange wedges.

29.   Walnuts and tofu crusted chicken

PREPARATION TIME: 15 minutes COOKING TIME: 15 minutes CALORIES: 370

INGREDIENTS FOR 2 SERVINGS

4 chicken breast slices 8 sage leaves 30 grams of chopped walnuts 20 grams of grated Tofu cheese 20 ml of coconut oil Salt and pepper to taste.

DIRECTIONS

Start with the chicken. Remove the excess fat and then if the slices are not thin enough, thin them with a meat mallet. Wash and dry the slices with absorbent paper and then sprinkle them on both sides with salt and pepper. Wash and dry the sage. Place 2 slices of chicken on a cutting board, place 2 sage leaves inside. Close the slices with the remaining slices, sealing them with toothpicks. Mix the walnuts with the grated tofu. Pass the slices over the walnuts and tofu cheese flour, pressing them to make the breading adhere well. Heat the coconut oil in a pan and as soon as it is hot, put the chicken to brown. Turn them over and cook until the meat is well cooked and golden on the outside. Serve the chicken immediately and hot, sprinkled with the cooking juices.

30. Pecans and tofu crusted turkey

PREPARATION TIME: 15 minutes COOKING TIME: 15 minutes CALORIES: 360

INGREDIENTS FOR 2 SERVINGS

4 slices of turkey breast 2 sage leaves 20 grams of chopped pecans 20 grams of grated Tofu cheese 10 ml of Olive oil Salt and pepper to taste.

DIRECTIONS

First, start with the turkey breast. Remove the excess fat and then if the slices are not thin enough, thin them with a meat mallet. Wash and dry the slices with a paper towel and then sprinkle them on both sides with salt and pepper. Wash and dry the sage. Place 2 slices of turkey on a cutting board, place 2 sage leaves inside. Close the slices with the remaining slices, sealing them with toothpicks. Mix the chopped pecans with the grated tofu cheese. Pass the slices over the pecans and tofu cheese flour, pressing them to make the breading adhere well. Heat the olive oil in a pan and as soon as it is hot, put the turkey to brown. Turn them over and cook until the meat is well cooked and golden on the outside. Serve the crusted turkey immediately and hot, sprinkled with the cooking juices.

31. Turkey and mushroom yogurt sauce

PREPARATION TIME: 15 minutes COOKING TIME: 25 minutes CALORIES: 295

INGREDIENTS FOR 2 SERVINGS

320 grams of turkey breast 150 grams of mushrooms 80 ml of soy yogurt ½ garlic clove 20 ml of olive oil 1 pinch of smoked paprika Salt to taste.

DIRECTIONS

Peel and wash the half garlic. Remove the earthy part of the mushrooms, wash them under running water, dry them and then cut them into slices. Clean the turkey breast, Remove excess fat and then cut into two slices. Wash it and dry it. Heat the olive oil in a pan. As soon as it is hot, brown the garlic and then remove it. Place the turkey slices and brown them on both sides until they are well cooked. Season with salt, pepper and mix of spices. Remove the turkey and keep it warm. Now add the mushrooms to the pan where you cooked the turkey. Brown them for 10 minutes and then add the soy yogurt. Stir to mix well, Let the sauce reduce and then season with salt and pepper. Add the turkey fillet, let it flavour and then turn off the heat. Serve the fillet sprinkled with the mushroom sauce.

32. Turkey breast with vegetables

PREPARATION TIME: 20 minutes COOKING TIME: 40 minutes CALORIES: 296

INGREDIENTS FOR 2 SERVINGS

400 grams of turkey breast 1 carrot 1 red onion 1 small yellow pepper 2 pickles a sprig of parsley 4 basil leaves 2 teaspoons of capers 1 tablespoon of apple cider vinegar olive oil to taste salt and pepper to taste

DIRECTIONS Wash and dry the turkey breast. Peel the carrot, wash it and cut it into small pieces. Peel the onion, wash it and cut it into slices. Put the carrot and half an onion in a pot with salted water. Bring to a boil and then put the turkey to cook for 40 minutes. Season with salt, pepper, and then turn off and put the turkey to drain. Peel and wash the garlic. Put it in the glass of the blender together with the capers, pine nuts and vinegar. Blend until you get a smooth cream. Now pour a spoonful of oil and blend for a few more seconds. Now cut the pepper in half, remove the seeds and white filaments, and then wash it. Cut it into thin sticks. Wash and dry the pickles and then cut into slices. Wash and dry the basil leaves and parsley and chop them. Now cut the turkey breast into slices and place the slices on serving plates. Now put the vegetables. Put the chopped aromatic herbs on top and then season with the caper sauce and serve.

33.   Baked salmon with green beans

PREPARATION TIME: 20 minutes COOKING TIME: 18 minutes CALORIES: 210

INGREDIENTS FOR 2 SERVINGS

300 grams of green beans 2 salmon fillets of 200 gr each half a lemon a sprig of thyme 1 sprig of parsley salt and pepper to taste olive oil to taste

DIRECTIONS

Wash the green beans and remove the tips. Boil some water with a little salt and then put the green beans to boil for 10 minutes. After 10 minutes, drain them and set aside. Wash and dry the salmon. Remove the bones if present. Wash the thyme sprig. Brush a pan with a little olive oil and put the green beans inside. Put the salmon fillets and the thyme sprig on top. Season everything with oil, salt, pepper, and lemon juice. Put in the oven and cook at 180 ° C for 8 minutes. After the cooking time, remove from the oven and let it rest for a couple of minutes. Put the salmon and green beans on serving plates, sprinkle everything with the cooking juices and serve.

34.   Salmon zucchini and mushrooms

PREPARATION TIME: 10 minutes COOKING TIME: 20 minutes CALORIES: 450

INGREDIENTS FOR 2 SERVINGs

2 salmon fillet (180 grams for each) 1 zucchini 150 grams of mushrooms 1 garlic clove ½ orange Two sprigs of rosemary Salt and Pepper To Taste.

DIRECTIONS

First, preheat the oven to 200° C. Start the recipe by cleaning the salmon fillet under running water, and drying it. Proceed, in the meantime, washing the zucchini. Clean the mushrooms too with a cloth, removing any soil. Cut the zucchini into slices and the mushrooms into 4 pieces. Peel and chop the garlic clove too. Spread some baking paper on a baking sheet. Place the vegetables in the centre of the pan. Place the salmon fillet on the side. Season fillets with salt and pepper. Squeeze the orange over it. Add the rosemary sprig. Close the parchment paper creating a sort of foil. Cook the tuna in a preheated oven for about 20 minutes. Always check the cooking of the fish, zucchini and mushrooms. You can serve when the fish and vegetables are cooked.

35. Orange salmon and vegetables

PREPARATION TIME: 20 minutes COOK TIME: 10 minutes
CALORIES: 450

INGREDIENTS FOR 2 SERVINGS 2 salmon filets of 150 grams each 1 zucchini 4 cherry tomatoes 1 lemon 120 ml of orange juice 1 tablespoon of dry thyme 1tsp of dry oregano 1 tablespoon of smoked paprika Salt and pepper to taste 2 tsp of olive oil

DIRECTIONS

Let us start by cleaning the salmon. Wash it under running water; remove it from the skin if present and if there are bones with fish tweezers. Rinse it quickly under running water and then dry it with paper towel. Sprinkle the fillets with a little salt and pepper and set aside. Now move on to the zucchini. Peel it, wash it under running water and then dry it. Now cut it into thin strip. Wash the cherry tomatoes, dry them and then cut them in half. In a small bowl, put together the orange juice, a tablespoon of olive oil and dried oregano, a pinch of salt and pepper. Mix well to mix everything. Take a pan large enough. Put the salmon in the pan and brush it with a little olive oil. Place the zucchini on the bottom. Sprinkle them with a pinch of salt. Now place the salmon fillet on top of the vegetables. Place the cherry tomatoes on top of the fillet and then sprinkle everything with the marinade. Sprinkle the thyme on top. Put the pan to bake in a preheated oven at 200 °C for 15 minutes. Check the cooking and, if necessary, continue cooking for another 5 minutes. Serve the orange salmon with the vegetables.

36. Sesame seeds salmon

PREPARATION TIME: 20 minutes COOK TIME: 8 minutes CALORIES: 480

INGREDIENTS FOR 2

2 salmon filets of 200 grams each 2 tsp of olive oil Salt and pepper to taste 1tsp of rosemary 1 lemon zest Sesame seed (white and black)

DIRECTIONS

Start the recipe by washing the filets of salmon under running water. 2   After washing and rinsing them, drain them and dry them with absorbent kitchen paper. 3   Salt and pepper the slices and place them in a pan suitable for the microwave oven. 4   Add the rosemary. 5   Cook the salmon at maximum power (800 watts) for 3 minutes. 6   If you are not satisfied with the cooking, cook for another minute. 7 Decorate with sesame seeds and serve.

37. Salmon fillet and cinnamon raspberries

PREPARATION TIME: 10 minutes + 1 hour freezer rest + 20 minutes marinating COOKING TIME: 10 minutes CALORIES: 320

INGREDIENTS FOR 2 SERVINGS

2 salmon fillets (150 grams for each) 3 tablespoon olive oil tsp smoked paprika Salt and pepper to taste. 1 tablespoon of orange juice 1 pinch of cinnamon 80 grams of raspberries

DIRECTIONS

First, chill the salmon fillets for at least an hour in the freezer. After the hour has passed, take them out, rinse them and let them dry well. In a small bowl, combine the spices. Mix the oil, paprika, salt and pepper well. Put the salmon in a large bowl and pour the marinade over it. Leave the fish to marinate for at least 20 minutes in the fridge. After twenty minutes, heat a pan with olive oil. Take the trout out of the fridge and cook it directly in the pan with the marinade. Cook the fish for 3 minutes on the side, taking care not to overcook it. While the fish is cooking, season the raspberries with the orange juice and a pinch of cinnamon. When the fish is ready, you can flake it and serve it on a serving dish. Accompanied by blueberries seasoned with orange juice and cinnamon.

38. Lime cod and cherry tomatoes

PREPARATION TIME: 15 minutes COOK TIME: 20/25 minutes CALORIES: 360

INGREDIENTS FOR 2 SERVINGS

2 cod filets of 200 grams each (already clean) 2 garlic cloves 1 small shallot 300 grams of cherry tomatoes 50 grams of green olives 100 ml of lime juice 1 tablespoon of oregano Salt and pepper to taste Olive oil to taste

DIRECTIONS Wash the cod fillets under tap water. Let them drain for a few minutes and dry them with kitchen paper. Peel the shallot, wash it and then chop it. Peel the garlic too, wash it and then chop it. Take a baking dish, brush it with a little oil and then lay the cod fillets on top. Drizzle with oil and sprinkle with the chopped garlic and shallot. Wash the cherry tomatoes, dry them and cut them in half. Spread the cherry tomatoes over the fish and sprinkle with salt, pepper and oregano. Finally, add the green olives. Place the pan inside the oven preheated to 200 ºC. Cook for about 20 minutes. After 10 minutes, turn the cod; sprinkle it with lime juice and then cook for another 10 minutes. Check the cooking and if they do not seem cooked enough, continue cooking for another 5 minutes. Serve the cod still warm.

39. Cod with citrus fruits

PREPARATION TIME: 15 minutes COOKING TIME: 30 minutes CALORIES: 240

INGREDIENTS FOR 2 SERVINGS 2 cod fillets of about 200 grams each Half a lemon Half an orange A sprig of fresh basil A sprig of parsley Salt to taste. Pepper as needed. Olive oil to taste **DIRECTIONS** Start by cleaning the cod fillets. Remove, if present, the excess bones with kitchen tweezers and then rinse the fillets under running water. Dry the fillets with parchment paper or a kitchen towel and set aside. Wash the parsley under running water and then chop finely. Remove the basil leaves from the stem and wash them under running water, then finely chop the leaves. Wash and slice the citrus fruits. Take aluminium foil large enough to hold both fillets. Brush the aluminium foil with a little olive oil. Salt and pepper the cod fillets on both sides. Place the cod fillets in the aluminium foil and then sprinkle a little oil over the fillets as well. Sprinkle the fish with basil, finely chopped parsley, and then put the lemon and orange cut into thin slices on top. Close the foil tightly and place it in a pan. Set the oven temperature to 180 degrees. Cook the cod for 30 minutes. After 10 minutes, take out the foil, being careful not to burn yourself, and blend with the juice of both citrus fruits Continue cooking at 180°C for another 20 minutes. Once out of the oven, remove the lemon and orange slices and serve the cod fillets.

40. Mint cod

PREPARATION TIME: 10 minutes COOKING TIME: 15 minutes CALORIES: 280

INGREDIENTS FOR 2 SERVINGS

400 grams of clean cod fillet 1 tablespoon of coconut oil 1 sprig of fresh mint 1 teaspoon of powdered ginger 1 teaspoon of lime zest Salt and pepper to taste.

DIRECTIONS

First, wash the cod fillet under running water, rinse it and let it dry Meanwhile, wash and chop the mint leaves. Once this is done, take the cod fillets and season with salt and pepper. Add the ginger powder and chopped mint. Place the cod fillets in a baking tray, sprinkle them with coconut oil, and grate the zest of a lime on top. Bake in the oven at 190 ° C for 15 minutes. When the mint cod fillets are cooked through, serve still hot.

41. Sea bass with lemon

PREPARATION TIME: 15 minutes COOKING TIME: 25 minutes CALORIES: 255

INGREDIENTS FOR 2 SERVINGS 2 sea bass fillets of about 150 grams each A lemon A sprig of fresh basil A sprig of parsley Salt and pepper to taste Olive oil to taste

DIRECTIONS Let us start by cleaning the sea bass fillets. Remove any excess bones with kitchen tweezers and then rinse the fillets under running water. Dry the fillets with a paper towel or kitchen towel and set aside. Wash the parsley under running water and then chop finely. Remove the basil leaves from the stem and wash them under running water, then finely chop the leaves. Take aluminium sheet large enough to hold both fillets. Brush the aluminium foil with a little olive oil. Salt and pepper the sea bass fillets on both sides. Place the sea bass fillets in aluminium foil and then sprinkle a little oil over the sea bass fillets as well. Sprinkle the sea bass with the finely chopped basil and parsley and then place the thinly sliced lemon on top. Close the foil tightly and place it in a baking pan. Preheat the oven to 180 °C and as soon as it is hot, cook the fish for about 20 minutes. If the sea bass is not completely cooked, continue cooking at 180 °C for another 5 minutes. Once out of the oven, remove the lemon slices and serve the sea bass fillets hot.

42.   Sea bass fillet with orange fennel

PREPARATION TIME: 15 minutes COOKING TIME: 15 minutes CALORIES: 220

INGREDIENTS FOR 2 SERVINGS

2 sea bass fillets already cut of 200 gr each 1 orange The inside of a fennel 1 tablespoon of orange juice Olive oil to taste Salt and pepper to taste.

DIRECTIONS Start by cleaning the sea bass fillets. Wash them under running water, check for bones. In this case, remove them with the help of kitchen tweezers. Rinse the sea bass quickly and then dry it with a kitchen towel or parchment paper. Cut the orange in half, wash it and cut one-half into thin slices. Wash and dry the internal parts of the fennel. In a small bowl, mix a tablespoon of oil, half a glass of water, and the orange juice. Now place the fish fillets in a baking dish or in a pan and season with a pinch of salt and a sprinkling of pepper. Cover the fish with the orange slices and the fennel. Pour the orange sauce over the fish. Cover the ovenproof dish or pan with aluminium foil and place in a preheated oven at 200° C for 15 minutes. You can serve the orange-scented fennels and fish.

43. Almonds Mediterranean sea bass

PREPARATION TIME: 15 minutes COOKING TIME: 10-15 minutes CALORIES: 230

INGREDIENTS FOR 2 SERVINGS

2 sea bass fillets already cut of 200 grams for each 12 cherry tomatoes 8 black olives 1 garlic clove 1 tablespoon of olive oil Salt and pepper to taste. 1 tablespoon of chopped almonds

DIRECTIONS

Start by cleaning the sea bass fillets. Wash them under running water, check if there are any bones. In this case, remove them with the help of kitchen tweezers. Quickly rinse the sea bass and then dry it with a kitchen towel or parchment paper. Spread 3 cherry tomatoes cut into fairly small pieces on each sea bass fillet. Add the pitted black olives cut into rounds (4 for each sea bass fillet). Also cut the garlic into pieces, distributing 1/2 clove on each fish fillet. Season with salt, add a sprinkling of oregano and sprinkle with a drizzle of olive oil. Bake the sea bass in a preheated oven at 180 ° C for 10-15 minutes, adjust the actual cooking minutes according to the power of your oven, and avoid overcooking the fish so as not to make it dry and stringy. Meanwhile, peel the almonds and chop them. Serve the sea bass with a sprinkling of chopped almonds.

SNACKS

44.   Fruit salad with dried fruit

PREPARATION TIME: 30 minutes CALORIES: 260

INGREDIENTS FOR 4 SERVINGS

1 apple 3 blood oranges 2 kiwis 10 hazelnuts 6 walnuts 20 grams of sliced almonds the juice of one lemon 1 teaspoon of cinnamon powder

DIRECTIONS

Peel the apple, wash it, remove the seeds, and then cut it into cubes. Peel the kiwis, cut them in half, remove the central part and then wash them. Cut them into cubes. Put apples and kiwis in a large bowl and season with lemon juice. Shell the walnuts and hazelnuts and then put them into the bowl with fruits. Also, add the sliced almonds. Peel 2 of the three oranges and cut them into wedges, then put them in the bowl together with the other fruits. Squeeze the other orange and sprinkle the other ingredients with the juice. Sprinkle everything with cinnamon, leave to flavour for 30 minutes, and then put the fruit salad in serving bowls and serve.

45.   Fruit salad with plums and melon

PREPARATION TIME: 20 minutes+2 hours resting in fridge
CALORIES: 161

INGREDIENTS FOR 2 SERVINGS

1 small melon 200 grams of prunes 1 teaspoon of stevia 50 ml
of unsweetened orange juice Chopped walnuts to taste

DIRECTIONS

Divide the melon in half and then peel it. Remove the seeds,
wash the pulp, and then cut it into cubes and put it in a bowl.
Wash the plums, divide them in half and then remove the
stones. Cut the plums into slices and then put them in the bowl
with the melon. Season with the orange juice and stevia, mix
gently and then refrigerate for 2 hours. After two hours, remove
the fruit salad from the fridge, put it in two bowls, garnish with
chopped walnuts and serve.

46. Fruit salad with strawberry sauce

PREPARATION TIME: 25 minutes CALORIES: 173

INGREDIENTS FOR 2 SERVINGS

half a melon 2 apricots 2 peaches 75 grams of blueberries 1
kiwi 100 grams of blackberries 100 grams of wild strawberries
1 lemon 1 teaspoon of stevia

DIRECTIONS

Start by preparing the strawberry sauce. Wash and dry the wild
strawberries, put in the blender glass with the lemon juice and
stevia. Blend at maximum speed until you get a fluid mixture.
Put the sauce to rest in the fridge until the other ingredients are
ready. Peel the melon and remove the seeds, wash the pulp, and
then cut it into cubes. Peel and wash the kiwis, then cut them
into small pieces. Peel the fish and apricots, remove the stone,
then wash and cut them into cubes. Wash and dry the
blackberries and blueberries. Collect all the fruit in a bowl.
Sprinkle the fruit with the strawberry sauce and then mix
gently. Now put the fruit salad in two individual bowls,
decorated with chopped dried fruit to taste, and serve.

47. Pineapple and strawberry fruit salad with mint

PREPARATION TIME: 20 minutes+ 30 minutes to rest in fridge CALORIES: 224

INGREDIENTS FOR 4 SERVINGS

Half a pineapple 400 grams of strawberries A small apple The juice of half a lemon A teaspoon of stevia 8 mint leaves 1 jar of soy yogurt A teaspoon of maple syrup A tablespoon of coconut milk

DIRECTIONS

Peel the pineapple, wash the pulp and then cut it into cubes. Peel the apple, cut it in half and remove the seeds. Wash it and then cut it into cubes. Put the fruit in a bowl. Wash and dry the mint leaves and put them in the bowl with the fruit. Season with lemon juice, stevia, and mix. In a small bowl, combine the yogurt, maple syrup and coconut milk. Mix until you get a homogeneous mixture. Finally wash and dry the strawberries and then cut them into slices. Put them in the bowl with the rest of the fruit. Now put the fruit salad to rest in the fridge for 30 minutes. After 30 minutes, take the fruit salad and put it in 4 bowls. Sprinkle them with the yogurt sauce and serve.

48. Detox smoothie

PREPARATION TIME: 10 minutes CALORIES: 93

INGREDIENTS FOR 2 SERVINGS

50 grams of spinach A stick of celery Half a cucumber 2 green apples 4 ice cubes

DIRECTIONS

Wash and dry the spinach. Peel the celery, wash it and cut it into small pieces. Wash the cucumber and cut it into small pieces. Cut the apples in half, remove the seeds and then wash them. Put all the ingredients in the blender glass. Add the ice and vanilla and blend everything at high speed. Blend until you get a thick and creamy mixture. Put the smoothie in the glasses, add the straws and serve.

49.   Smoothie bowl with kiwi and spinach

PREPARATION TIME: 10 minutes CALORIES: 227

INGREDIENTS FOR 2 SERVINGS

4 kiwis 6 mint leaves 100 grams of spinach 2 pots of soy yogurt Pumpkin seeds to taste Chopped pistachio to taste Chia seeds to taste Almond flakes to taste

DIRECTIONS

Wash and dry the spinach. Peel the kiwis, wash them and then cut them in half. Wash and dry the mint leaves. Put kiwi, mint, spinach and yogurt in the blender glass. Blend everything until you get a thick and creamy mixture. Put the mixture in two bowls. Decorate with chia seeds, almonds, pistachio and pumpkin seeds and serve.

50.   Peach smoothie

PREPARATION TIME: 10 minutes CALORIES: 144

INGREDIENTS FOR 2 SERVINGS

4 peaches 4 ice cubes 1 teaspoon of stevia 100 grams of soy
yogurt 1 tsp ground cinnamon

DIRECTIONS

Peel the peaches, wash them, remove the stone and then cut
them into small pieces. Put the peaches in the glass of the
blender. Add the yogurt, cinnamon, stevia and turn on the
blender. Blend for 30 seconds and then add the ice cubes.
Blend again until you get a thick and homogeneous smoothie.
Distribute the smoothie in the glasses, decorate with a little
ground cinnamon, place the straws and serve.

51. Ginger and melon smoothie

PREPARATION TIME: 10 minutes CALORIES: 51

INGREDIENTS FOR 2 SERVINGS

3 slices of melon 1 tablespoon of fresh grated ginger 6 ice cubes 100 ml of unsweetened almond milk A teaspoon of vanilla essence A teaspoon of stevia.

DIRECTIONS

Peel the melon slices, wash them and then cut them into cubes. Put the melon in the glass of the blender and add the almond milk, stevia, ginger and vanilla. Blend for a minute and then add the ice cubes. Blend again until you get a smooth and homogeneous smoothie. Distribute the smoothie in two glasses; place the straws, decorated with mint leaves and serve.

52. Peach and apricot smoothie

PREPARATION TIME: 10 minutes CALORIES: 87

INGREDIENTS FOR 2 SERVINGS

2 peaches 4 apricots 150 ml of unsweetened almond milk 1 teaspoon of stevia a teaspoon of ground cinnamon 4 ice cubes

DIRECTIONS

Peel the peaches and apricots, wash them, cut them in half and remove the stone. Put the peaches and apricots in the glass of the blender. Add the almond milk, cinnamon, stevia and ice cubes. Blend everything at maximum speed until you get a thick and homogeneous mixture. Distribute the smoothie in two glasses, decorate with chopped pistachios, add the straws and serve.

53. Watermelon and tofu skewers

PREPARATION TIME: 10 minutes CALORIES: 163

INGREDIENTS FOR 2 SERVINGS

1 slice of watermelon 200 grams of tofu 1 lemon 1 sprig of thyme Olive oil to taste Salt and pepper to taste

DIRECTIONS

Peel the watermelon. Try to eliminate all the seeds without damaging the pulp and then cut it into cubes. Dab the tofu with absorbent paper and then cut it into cubes of the same size as the watermelon. Take a skewer and put first a cube of feta and then one of watermelon. Proceed in this way until you have used up all the ingredients. Wash and dry the thyme and then remove only the leaves. Put in a bowl, oil, salt, pepper and the thyme leaves and mix well. Sprinkle the skewers with the emulsion, put them on serving plates and serve.

54. Avocado and tomato tartare

PREPARATION TIME: 15 minutes CALORIES: 228

INGREDIENTS FOR 2 SERVINGS

1 avocado 2 tomatoes 1 lemon 1 shallot olive oil to taste salt
and pepper to taste chives to taste

DIRECTIONS

Peel and wash the avocado. Cut it in half, remove the stone and
then cut it into cubes. Put the avocado in a bowl and season it
with the lemon juice. Wash the tomatoes and then cut them
into cubes. Peel the onion, wash it and cut it into small pieces.
Put the tomatoes and onion in the bowl with the avocado.
Season with oil, salt, pepper, and mix. To serve, put the
ingredients in two glasses, decorate with chopped chives and
serve.

55.   Avocado and berries smoothie

PREPARATION TIME: 15 minutes CALORIES: 258

INGREDIENTS FOR 2 SERVINGS

100 grams of mixed berries 1 avocado A teaspoon of honey
The juice of half a lemon 2 teaspoons of grated ginger 300 ml
of coconut milk 4 ice cubes

DIRECTIONS

Peel and wash the avocado. Cut it in half, remove the stone and
then cut it into slices. Wash and dry the berries. Put the berries
and the avocado in the glass of the blender and blend them for a
few seconds. Now add the coconut milk, lemon juice, ginger
and honey and blend again for another 30 seconds. Now add
the ice cubes and blend until you get a thick and velvety
mixture. Divide the shake into glasses, add the straws, decorate
with mint leaves and serve.

56.   Avocado and strawberry fruit salad

PREPARATION TIME: 15 minutes+30 minutes to rest in fridge
CALORIES: 225

INGREDIENTS FOR 2 SERVINGS

1 avocado 100 grams of strawberries Half a lemon Chopped pistachios 50 ml of unsweetened orange juice A teaspoon of honey

DIRECTIONS

Peel and wash the avocado. Cut it in half, remove the stone and then cut it into cubes. Wash the strawberries and then cut them into slices. Put the avocado and strawberries in a bowl. In a bowl, mix the orange juice, the filtered lemon juice and the honey. Season the avocado and strawberries with the emulsion and then refrigerate to rest for 30 minutes. After the resting time, divide the fruit salad into two bowls, decorated with chopped pistachios and serve.

57.Pear and almond smoothie

PREPARATION TIME: 10 minutes CALORIES: 232

INGREDIENTS FOR 2 SERVINGS

2 small pears 40 grams of peeled almonds 1 soy yogurt 60 ml of coconut milk 4 ice cubes 1 teaspoon of vanilla essence

DIRECTIONS

Peel the pears, wash them, cut them in half and remove the seeds. Put the pears and almonds in the glass of the mixer, together with the yogurt, vanilla and coconut milk. Blend everything at high speed for a minute and then add the ice cubes. Continue to blend until you get a thick and homogeneous smoothie. Put the smoothie in the glasses, put on the straws and serve.

58.   Pear and peach smoothie

PREPARATION TIME: 10 minutes CALORIES: 153

INGREDIENTS FOR 2 SERVINGS

2 pears 2 peaches 1 lemon 1 teaspoon of vanilla essence 100 ml of unsweetened almond milk 4 ice cubes

DIRECTIONS

Peel and wash the peaches and pears. Cut the peaches in half, remove the stone and then put them in the glass of the blender. Cut the pears in half, remove the seeds, and then put them in the blender. Add the filtered lemon juice, vanilla and almond milk and blend for 1 minute. Add the ice cubes and blend for another minute. Divide the smoothie into two glasses, put on the straws and serve.

59.   Granola with amaranth and oats

PREPARATION TIME: 10 minutes COOKING TIME: 30 minutes CALORIES: 276

INGREDIENTS FOR 2 SERVINGS

30 grams of almonds 30 grams of walnuts 30 grams of hazelnuts 30 grams of pistachios 20 grams of amaranth flakes 40 grams of rolled oats A spoonful of Goji berries 2 tablespoons of maple syrup

DIRECTIONS

Put the dried fruit in the glass of the mixer and chop everything finely. Put the chopped dried fruit in a bowl together with the amaranth and oat flakes. Add the goji berries and the maple syrup and mix everything well. Take a baking sheet and cover it with parchment paper. Roll out the dough along the parchment paper and cook at 160 ° C for 30 minutes. After the cooking time, take the granola out of the oven, let it cool and then break it with your hands. Put the granola in the bowls and serve.

60. Melon salad

PREPARATION TIME: 15 minutes CALORIES: 141

INGREDIENTS FOR 2 SERVINGS

1 melon 100 grams of watermelon 100 grams of strawberries 50 ml of unsweetened orange juice a teaspoon of vanilla powder coconut grains to taste

DIRECTIONS

Cut the melon in half. Remove the seeds and peel it. Wash it and then cut it into cubes. Peel the watermelon, remove the seeds and cut it into cubes. Wash the strawberries and then cut them into slices. Put the fruit in a bowl and sprinkle with vanilla. Add the orange juice and mix gently. Transfer the fruit salad to the fridge for 30 minutes. After 30 minutes, remove the fruit salad from the fridge, put it in the bowls, sprinkle it with coconut grains and serve.

61. Lime and ginger sorbet

PREPARATION TIME: 15 minutes CALORIES: 44

INGREDIENTS FOR 2 SERVINGS

2 limes A tablespoon of grated ginger 3 teaspoons of honey
200 grams of ice

DIRECTIONS

Peel the limes and remove only the pulp. Wash the zest and keep it aside. Put the lime pulp, ginger and honey in the blender glass. Blend everything at high speed for one minute. Now add the ice and blend until you get a homogeneous mixture. Put the sorbet in the glasses, decorate with the lime zest and serve.

62.   Peach and carrot smoothie

PREPARATION TIME: 15 minutes CALORIES: 66

INGREDIENTS FOR 2 SERVINGS

2 peaches The juice of one lemon 1 carrot 1 teaspoon of stevia
6 ice cubes

DIRECTIONS

Peel the carrot, wash it and cut it into small pieces. Peel the
peaches, wash them, cut them in half, remove the stone and
then cut them into pieces. Put the carrots and peaches in the
glass of the blender. Add the lemon juice, stevia and ice cubes.
Blend on high speed until you get a thick and smooth smoothie.
Put the smoothie in the glasses, add the straws and serve.

63. Vegan Golden Milk

PREPARATION TIME: 15 minutes CALORIES: 123

INGREDIENTS FOR 2 SERVINGS

400 ml of unsweetened almond milk 1 tablespoon of ground cinnamon 2 teaspoons of coconut oil 35 grams of turmeric powder 10 grams of ginger powder A spoonful of maple syrup A pinch of black pepper

DIRECTIONS

Mix the coconut oil with the turmeric, cinnamon, ginger and black pepper in a saucepan; add 150 ml of water and cook over low heat, turning the mixture, until a sort of elastic dough forms. Heat the almond milk in a saucepan. Add the spice paste and let it melt over moderate heat. Add the maple syrup, stir again and turn off. Serve immediately the golden milk vegan.

64.   Smoothie bowl with apples, banana, and carrots

PREPARATION TIME: 15 minutes CALORIES: 298

INGREDIENTS FOR 2 SERVINGS

2 red apples 2 medium sized carrots 1 banana a tablespoon of soy yogurt a teaspoon of grated ginger a tablespoon of orange juice a teaspoon of stevia 20 grams of flaked almonds 1 teaspoon of chia seeds

DIRECTIONS

Peel the apples, cut them in half and remove the seeds. Wash them and then cut them into small pieces. Put the apples in the bowl and season with the orange juice. Peel and wash the carrot, then cut it into small pieces. Peel the banana and then cut it into small pieces. Now put the fruit and carrots in the glass of the blender, and add the yogurt, ginger and stevia. Blend everything at high speed until you get a thick and homogeneous mixture. Put the mixture in two bowls. Now take a pan and toast the chia seeds and almonds for a couple of minutes. Season the smoothie with the almond and chia crumble and serve.

65.　Mint and cherries smoothie

PREPARATION TIME: 10 minutes CALORIES: 81

INGREDIENTS FOR 2 SERVINGS

6 cherries A banana 2 mint leaves A teaspoon of stevia 6 ice cubes 100 ml of unsweetened almond milk

DIRECTIONS

Wash the cherries, cut them in half and remove the stone. Peel the banana and cut it into small pieces. Wash and dry the mint leaves. Put the banana, cherries and mint in the blender glass. Add the stevia, almond milk, and ice cubes and blend everything at high speed. Blend until you get a thick and smooth smoothie. Put the smoothie in the glasses, add the straws and serve.

DINNER RECIPES

66. Beef burger with almonds, rocket salad and green beans

PREPARATION TIME: 20 minutes+ 30 minutes to rest in fridge COOKING TIME: 20 minutes CALORIES: 378

INGREDIENTS FOR 2 SERVINGS

2 beef burgers of 150 grams each 100 grams of green beans 25 grams of rocket 1 clove of garlic 20 grams of almond flakes 1 orange Olive oil to taste Salt and pepper to taste

DIRECTIONS Wash and dry the orange. Cut it in half. Squeeze the juice of half-orange and cut the other half into rings. Peel the garlic, wash it and then mash it. Put the garlic, a little salt, pepper, and the orange juice in a bowl. Now put the burgers in the bowl and put them to marinate for 30 minutes in the fridge. In the meantime, prepare the green beans. Tick them and then wash them. Cook them in abundant salted water for 15 minutes. Drain and set aside. Wash and dry the rocket. Toast the almonds for two minutes in a non-stick pan. Now heat a grill and as soon as it is hot, grill the burgers for 3 minutes per side. Take two serving plates and put the orange slices on the bottom. Put the burgers on top, spread the rocket and green beans on top and season with oil, salt, and pepper. Sprinkle with toasted almonds and serve.

67. Beef with asparagus

PREPARATION TIME: 12 minutes COOKING TIME: 20 minutes CALORIES: 360

INGREDIENTS FOR 2 SERVINGS

2 beef fillet (150 grams about for each) 200 grams of asparagus 25 ml of olive oil 1 pinch of salt 1 tsp powdered ginger ¼ tsp smoked paprika

DIRECTIONS

First, wash the asparagus well. Remove the white part of the stem and keep the more tender tips aside. Now you can take the beef fillet and rinse it under running water. Dry it well with a paper towel. Wash and dry beef fillet too. Season beef fillet with salt and pepper. Season further with ginger powder and smoked paprika. Lightly oil a baking pan and place the asparagus first and then the beef fillet. Bake in a preheated oven at 190° C for about 15/20 minutes. Check both the doneness of both meat and asparagus. When all it is done serve the beef fillet still warm with the asparagus.

68. Orange beef and veggies

PREPARATION TIME: 10 minutes COOKING TIME: 20 minutes CALORIES: 450

INGREDIENTS FOR 2 SERVINGS

2 beef fillet (200 grams about for each) ½ teaspoon of onion powder ½ zucchini 150 grams of mushrooms 12 cherry tomatoes 1 garlic clove ½ orange 10 ml of coconut oil Two sprigs of thyme Salt and Pepper To Taste.

DIRECTIONS First, preheat the oven to 200°C. Start the recipe by cleaning the beef fillet under running water, and drying it. Proceed, in the meantime, washing the half zucchini. Clean the mushrooms too with a cloth, removing any soil. Cut the zucchini into slices and the mushrooms into 4 pieces. Wash and halve cherry tomatoes. Peel and chop the garlic clove too. Spread some baking paper on a baking sheet. Place the vegetables in the centre of the pan. Place beef fillets on the side. Season meat with salt, pepper and onion powder. Squeeze the orange over it and drip the liquid coconut oil. Add the thyme sprig. Close the parchment paper creating a sort of foil. Cook the meat in a preheated oven for about 15 minutes. Always check the cooking of the beef and vegetables If it is still not ready, keep on cooking for about 5 minutes. You can serve when beef fillet and vegetables are cooked.

69. Beef with cabbage

PREPARATION TIME: 5 minutes COOKING TIME: 35/40 minutes CALORIES: 360

INGREDIENTS FOR 2 SERVINGS

300 grams of beef fillet 200 grams of green cabbage Half a spring onion 2 juniper berries 1 bay leaf 15 ml of olive oil 40 ml of beef broth Salt and pepper to taste.

DIRECTIONS Start with the meat. Remove the excess fat then wash and dry it. Place the rack on a sheet of aluminium foil, brush the meat with a little olive oil and then close the aluminium foil. Place the meat on a baking sheet. Bake in the oven at 180° C for 20 minutes about. Meanwhile, prepare the cabbage. Peel, wash and then finely chop the spring onion. Wash the cabbage, dry it and then cut it into thin slices. Wash and dry the bay leaves. In a pan, put a drizzle of oil to heat. When the oil is hot, sauté onion chopped for a couple of minutes, stirring constantly to keep it from burning. Now add the cabbage, season with salt and pepper and mix. After a couple of minutes, add the bay leaf, juniper berries and broth. Cook for 30 minutes, adding water if necessary, and stirring occasionally. As soon as the beef is cooked, remove it from the oven, let the meat rest for 5 minutes and then slice it. Put the cabbage on the bottom of the serving dish, then over beef slices and sprinkle everything with the cooking juices of the cabbage.

70. Beef and fennels

PREPARATION TIME: 15 minutes COOKING TIME: 15 minutes CALORIES: 360

INGREDIENTS FOR 2 SERVINGS

2 beef fillets (150 grams about for each) 5 grams of smoked paprika 1 pinch of chilli powder ½ cup fennels ½ lemon 20 ml of olive oil Salt and pepper to Taste.

DIRECTIONS Start with the fennels. Remove the inner part, separate the various leaves, wash them under running water, dry them and then cut the fennel into slices. Also, wash some pieces of fennel and set them aside. Take a pan and heat half a tablespoon of oil. Let the oil heat up and then put the fennel slices for about ten minutes to sauté, adding salt and a drop of water. Now switch to the beef fillet. Wash it under running water and let it dry. Now take a pan and put 2 sheets of parchment paper inside the pan. Grease the parchment paper with a little oil, add the beef, salt it, and sprinkle it with chilli powder and paprika. Then sprinkle beef with lemon juice and a drizzle of olive oil and the fennel pieces that you had set aside. Put the beef in a preheated oven at 190° F for about 15 minutes. As soon as they are ready, remove the beef fillet from the parchment paper, remove the fennel pieces too and place beef in a serving dish surrounded by previously cooked fennel. Serve still hot.

71. Beef and avocado

PREPARATION TIME: 10 minutes COOKING TIME: 20 minutes CALORIES: 460

INGREDIENTS FOR 2 SERVINGS

2 beef fillet (200 grams for each) 20 ml of coconut oil 1 lime 1 avocado 1/2 spring onion 1 tsp chives 1 tsp smoked paprika Salt and pepper to taste A sprig of chopped parsley

DIRECTIONS

Peel the avocado, remove the stone, then wash, and dry it. Cut it into cubes. Peel and wash the spring onion. Dry it and then chop it. Wash and dry the fillet and then cut it into small pieces. Wash and dry the lime, grate the peel and set it aside and then squeeze the pulp and strain the juice into a bowl. Put the meat, salt, pepper, chives, coconut oil, paprika, and parsley in the bowl with the lime juice. Stir gently to mix everything. Let sauté the beef filet with the sauce for few minutes in a pan. When it will be done, serve the meat in the centre of the plate. Add the avocado cubes and serve.

72. Spicy chicken and broccoli

PREPARATION TIME: 10 minutes COOKING TIME: 20 minutes CALORIES: 380

INGREDIENTS FOR 2 SERVINGS

400 grams of Chicken breast 10 broccoli tops 4 grams of chilli powder 2 grams of ginger powder 1sprigs of rosemary ½ lime juice 10 ml of coconut oil Salt and pepper to taste

DIRECTIONS

Wash and dry the tops of the broccoli, then cut them into many pieces. Remove any bones and excess fat from the chicken, then wash and dry it. Wash and dry the rosemary. Put the coconut oil, lime, salt, chilli and ginger powder, and pepper in a bowl and mix with a fork until you get a homogeneous emulsion. Take one sheet of aluminium foil and place the chicken. Add the broccoli, rosemary, and then wet everything with the oil, and lime emulsion. Close the foil making sure to seal it well. Put in the oven and cook at 200°C for 20/22 minutes. When it is ready, remove the rosemary and serve the chicken with the broccoli, and sprinkled with the marinating liquid.

73.   Chicken broccoli roulade

PREPARATION TIME: 30 minutes + 30 minutes of rest in the fridge COOKING TIME: 40 minutes CALORIES: 390

INGREDIENTS FOR 2 SERVINGS

350 grams of whole chicken breast 150 grams of broccoli flowers 50 grams of cubed tofu 10 ml of olive oil Salt and pepper to Taste.

DIRECTIONS

 Wash the broccoli flowers under running water and then dry them. Then put them in a pot with water and salt and cook for 20 minutes. While broccoli florets are cooking, take the chicken breast, remove the bones and fat and then cut it horizontally in half. Beat it with a meat mallet to soften and thin it, then sprinkle it on both sides with salt and pepper. When the broccoli is cooked, drain it, let it cool and then cut it into small pieces. Take a sheet of cling film and place the bacon slices on top. Place the chicken breast on top. Place the broccoli first and then the tofu cubed inside the chicken. Roll up everything, using the plastic wrap and let it rest in the fridge for 30 minutes. Meanwhile, preheat the oven to 180° C. Brush a pan with olive oil and lie inside the roll. Cook for 30 minutes, adding a little water if necessary. Remove from the oven, let it rest for 5 minutes and then cut the roll into slices and serve.

74. Chicken and bell peppers

PREPARATION TIME: 15 minutes COOKING TIME: 10 minutes CALORIES: 360

INGREDIENTS FOR 2 SERVINGS

350 grams of chicken breast, cut into thin steaks about ¼-inch thick ½ teaspoon of salt, divided 20 ml of olive oil, divided ½ spring onion sliced ½ red bell pepper, cut into strips ½ yellow bell pepper, cut into strips 1 pinch of smoked paprika 1 pinch of black pepper 5 ml of apple cider wine vinegar 5 grams of Chopped fresh parsley

DIRECTIONS

Start by washing, removing seeds and slicing both bell peppers. Wash and chop spring onion. Now, season the chicken. To prevent overcrowding the skillet, which will inhibit browning, split the chicken in half and cook it in two batches. Sear half of it in the skillet in the oil. Reduce heat under the skillet and repeat with the second half of the chicken adding more oil. Take the chicken out of the skillet and set both batches on a plate with foil over it. Now, sauté the peppers and onion in a pan. Add both to the skillet and cook them. Stir them often and cook them until they are tender and starting to brown. Before adding any liquid, add the Italian seasoning and pepper to bloom the spices in the hot oil. They will become fragrant within about 30 seconds. Add in the vinegar and let it evaporate. Finish Cooking the chicken in the Sauce Now add the chicken back into the skillet with any accumulated juices from the plate and bring it all up to a simmer. Then just simmer on medium-low heat to thicken the sauce and cook the chicken all the way through. Serve still hot.

75.Avocado orange chicken

PREPARATION TIME: 5 minutes + 15 minutes of marinating in the fridge COOKING TIME: 10 minutes CALORIES: 460

INGREDIENTS FOR 2 SERVINGS

400 grams of chicken slices 1/2 orange ½ shallot 100 grams of cherry tomatoes ½ avocado ½ tsp dried thyme 1 pinch of smoked paprika Salt to taste Olive oil to taste

DIRECTIONS Wash and dry the chicken slices. Transfer the chicken to a large pan and season with oil, salt and paprika. Strain the juice from the orange, then sprinkle the chicken slices. Also, add the dried thyme and mix the slices to flavour them well. Cover with transparent paper and put them in the fridge for 15 minutes to marinate. Wash and dry the cherry tomatoes and then cut them into cubes. Peel the half shallot, wash it and chop it. Peel the half avocado, remove the stone, wash it, dry it and then cut it into cubes. Put the tomatoes, avocado, and shallot in a bowl, season with oil, salt, pepper, and mix to mix everything. After 15 minutes, remove the chicken from the fridge. Heat a grill, which should be hot, and cook the slices for 3/4 minutes per side. The chicken should be well cooked and have grill streaks on the surface. Transfer the chicken to a serving plate and garnish with the avocado and cherry tomato mixture.

76.   Mushroom chicken thighs

PREPARATION TIME: 10 minutes COOKING TIME: 15 minutes CALORIES: 400

INGREDIENTS FOR 2 SERVINGS

4 skinless chicken thighs ½ orange juice 1 garlic clove minced ½ tsp dried thyme ½ tsp Salt 1 pinch of chilli powder 1 tablespoon olive oil ½ cup sliced mushrooms 1 tsp mustard 20 grams of tofu cheese 1 tsp fresh parsley chopped 1 tsp dried rosemary ½ cup vegetal cooking Cream Salt and black pepper to taste

DIRECTIONS

Pat chicken thighs dry with paper towel and trim off excess fat. Season the chicken thighs with orange juice and salt. Let it absorb the juice for 10 minutes. Peel and mince the garlic clove. Combine the garlic clove, thyme, rosemary, and pepper. Coat the chicken evenly with the combined seasoning. Heat 1 tablespoon of oil a large pan or skillet over medium-high heat and sear chicken thighs in batches until browned on each side and no longer pink in centre (about 8 minutes each side, depending on thickness). Transfer to a plate; set aside and keep warm. Meanwhile, prepare mushrooms cream. On the same pan or skillet, put the olive oil and add the mushrooms. Season with salt, pepper, and cook until soft (about 3 minutes). Add the garlic, parsley, and rosemary; sauté until fragrant (about 1 minute). Add the mustard teaspoon too, then stir in vegetal cooking cream, bring to a simmer, then reduce heat and continue cooking until sauce has thickened slightly. Stir in the tofu cheese and allow it to melt through the sauce for a further 4 minutes, while occasionally stirring. Return chicken to the pan. Taste test and season with salt and pepper to your taste. Serve immediately.

77.Almond chicken with olives and mushrooms

PREPARATION TIME: 20 minutes COOKING TIME: 20 minutes CALORIES: 420

INGREDIENTS FOR 2 SERVINGS

350 grams of chicken breast 150 grams of mushrooms 8 pitted black olives 20 grams of almond flour 30 ml of chicken broth 1 garlic clove 20 ml of olive oil Salt and pepper to taste.

DIRECTIONS

Start with cleaning the mushrooms. Remove the earthy part, rinse them quickly under running water and then dry them. Cut them into thin slices. Peel and wash the garlic. Switch to the chicken. Remove any residues of skin, fat and bones and then cut it into many thin strips. Take a plate, put the almond flour and flour the chicken strips. After the operation, keep the chicken slices aside. Put the olive oil in a pan and as soon as it is hot, add the garlic. Fry it until completely pierced and then add the mushrooms. Cook the mushrooms over medium heat for 10 minutes, seasoning with salt and pepper, then remove the garlic and add the chicken. Cook for another 8 minutes, adding a little chicken broth from time to time. After 8 minutes, add the olives and cook for another two minutes, seasoning with salt and pepper. Remove the chicken from the pan and place it with the mushrooms and olives on two serving plates. Stir in the cooking juices of the chicken, reduce it and then sprinkle the chicken with the sauce.

78. Tofu turkey and veggies

PREPARATION TIME: 15 minutes COOKING TIME: 15 minutes CALORIES: 480

INGREDIENTS FOR 2 SERVINGS

400 grams of turkey breast 10 ml of coconut oil 100 grams of broccoli florets 150 grams of spinach 100 grams of shredded tofu cheese 20 ml of soy yogurt 1 pinch of Italian seasoning Salt and pepper to taste 2 garlic cloves minced

DIRECTIONS

Begin by wash and dry the turkey breast, then cut it into slices. Meanwhile, wash broccoli taking only florets. Wash spinach leaves too. Peel and mince garlic cloves. Heat 1 tablespoon of coconut oil in a large saucepan over medium-high heat. Add the sliced turkey slices, season with Italian seasoning, salt & pepper. Sauté for 4-5 minutes or until turkey meat is golden and cooked through.   Add the garlic and sauté for another minute or until fragrant. Add broccoli florets, spinach leaves, shredded tofu cheese, and soy yogurt. Cook for another 3-4 minutes or until the broccoli is cooked through. Serve still hot.

79.   Turkey with tomatoes and bell peppers

PREPARATION TIME: 15 minutes COOKING TIME: 10 minutes CALORIES: 360

INGREDIENTS FOR 2 SERVINGS

350 grams of turkey breast 1 teaspoon salt, divided 30 ml of olive oil, divided ½ shallot sliced 1 red bell pepper, cut into strips 1 yellow bell pepper, cut into strips 1 pinch of Italian seasoning 1 pinch of black pepper 20 ml of apple cider vinegar 14-ounce can crushed tomatoes 10 grams of chopped fresh parsley

DIRECTIONS

Start by washing, removing seeds and slicing both bell peppers. Wash and chop shallot. Now, season the turkey. To prevent overcrowding the skillet, which will inhibit browning, split the turkey in half and cook it in two batches. Sear half of it in the skillet in the oil. Reduce heat under the skillet and repeat with the second half of the turkey adding more oil. Take the turkey out of the skillet and set both batches on a plate with foil over it. Now, sauté the peppers and shallot in a pan. Add both to the skillet and cook them. Stir them often and cook them until they are tender and starting to brown. Before adding any liquid, add the Italian seasoning and pepper to bloom the spices in the hot oil. They will become fragrant within about 30 seconds. Add in the vinegar and let it evaporate. Add tomatoes and simmer. Finish Cooking the Turkey in the Sauce Now add the turkey back into the skillet with any accumulated juices from the plate and bring it all up to a simmer. Then just simmer on medium-low heat to thicken the sauce and cook the turkey all the way through

80. Turkey and vegetable salad

PREPARATION TIME: 15 minutes COOKING TIME: 25 minutes CALORIES: 300

INGREDIENTS FOR 2 SERVINGS

300 grams of turkey breast 100 grams of lettuce 50 grams of cherry tomatoes 100 grams of avocado 1 sprig of rosemary 2 sage leaves Dried oregano to taste Salt and pepper to taste. Two tablespoons apple cider vinegar

DIRECTIONS

Wash and dry sage and rosemary. Take the turkey breast, remove any fat, skin and bones and then wash it under running water. Dry it and divide it in half. Take a pot, put 100 ml of water, add salt and bring it to a boil. Place a steamer basket or alternatively a large colander on the pot. Place the turkey, sage and rosemary in the basket. Cook for 25 minutes, seasoning with salt and pepper. After the cooking time, turn off and let the meat cool. Meanwhile, wash and dry the lettuce and then cut it into thin strips. Wash and dry the cherry tomatoes and cut them in half. Peel the avocado, remove the stone, wash it under running water and dry it with absorbent paper. Cut it into cubes. Take a salad bowl and put a pinch of salt and pepper inside the vegetables and mix. Take the turkey, which has cooled in the meantime, and cut it into cubes. Put it in the salad bowl together with the vegetables. Season the salad with olive oil and apple cider vinegar, season with salt, pepper if necessary, and then serve.

81.Pecans and tofu crusted salmon

PREPARATION TIME: 15 minutes COOKING TIME: 15 minutes CALORIES: 420

Ingredients for 2 SERVINGs 2

salmon fillets of 150 grams for each 2 sage leaves 1 tablespoon chopped pecans 1 tsp grated Tofu cheese 1 tablespoon Olive oil Salt and pepper to taste.

DIRECTIONS First, start with the salmon fillet. Remove the skin and then wash it very well. Dry salmon fillet with a paper towel. Now you can cut salmon fillets into slices. After that, sprinkle them on both sides with salt and pepper. Wash and dry the sage. Place 2 slices of salmon on a cutting board, place 1 sage leaves inside. Close the slices with the remaining slices, sealing them with toothpicks. Mix the chopped pecans with the grated Parmesan. Pass the slices over the pecans and tofu cheese, pressing them to make the breading adhere well. Heat the olive oil in a pan and as soon as it is hot, put the salmon to brown. Turn them over and cook until the fish is well cooked and golden on the outside. Serve the crusted salmon immediately and hot, sprinkled with the cooking juices.

82. Almond crusted salmon

PREPARATION TIME: 15 minutes + 1 hour of rest in the freezer
COOKING TIME: 5/6 minutes CALORIES: 370

INGREDIENTS FOR 2 SERVINGS 2 salmon fillets of 150 grams or each 50 grams of chopped almonds 1 and ½ tablespoon of coconut oil 1 pinch of Italian seasoning Salt and pepper to taste **DIRECTIONS** Start by putting the salmon fillet in the freezer for at least an hour so that as soon as it comes out of the freezer it will be easier to cut it into fillets without breaking the fibres. After the hour, remove the fish from the freezer, rinse it and dry it with absorbent paper. Cut it lengthwise to obtain slices. Try not to cut too thick slices. Put the salmon slices in a baking tray and sprinkle them with a little coconut oil. Season salmon slices with Italian seasoning, salt and pepper. If you do not have ground almonds, you can take them whole and chop them yourself. Take the slices of salmon and pass them in the almond breading making sure to press well so that it is breaded on all sides. Put a tablespoon of coconut oil in a non-stick pan and let it heat up. As soon as the oil starts to sizzle, place the breaded fish slices in the pan and cook them for a couple of minutes on both sides. Cook until the salmon has just turned a lighter pink or it would be overcooked. As soon as the slices of breaded salmon with almonds are cooked, place it on a serving dish and serve.

83. Salmon burger

PREPARATION TIME: 15 minutes COOKING TIME: 15 minutes CALORIES: 360

INGREDIENTS FOR 2 SERVINGS

For Salmon burger: 200 grams of skinless salmon fillet 15 grams of tofu grated cheese ½ red onion. 1 tablespoon fresh dill For the sauce: 100 grams of soy yogurt 20 grams of mustard 1 tablespoon of fresh dill cut off. 2 new chives teaspoons, hacked.

DIRECTIONS

Start by washing and cutting dill and chives. Meanwhile prepare the sauce combining soy yogurt, dill, mustard and chives in a little mug. Set aside. Wash and dry salmon fillet, than cut it into 1 1/2 inch cubes and transfer to a food processor. Peel wash and chop red onion. Mix and ground salmon cubes. Add tofu cheese, onion and fresh dill. Forms 4 burgers. Through the frying pan and heat the pan with tiny quantities of olive oil. Cook burgers until browned for 3-4 minutes. Cook until browned for another 3-4 minutes. Serve with soy yogurt and dill sauce.

84.   Salmon and avocado salad

PREPARATION TIME: 15 minutes CALORIES: 480

INGREDIENTS FOR 2 SERVINGS

200 grams of smoked salmon 1 avocado 2 tablespoon soy sauce 2 tsp ginger powder 1 tsp garlic powder 1 tsp rice vinegar 1 cucumber 1 tablespoon olive oil Sesame seeds

DIRECTIONS

Start by taking smoke salmon and cut into slices. Meanwhile, prepare the marinade. In a small bowl, pour the olive oil, soy sauce, rice vinegar, and ginger and garlic powder. After that take the salmon slices and put them in a bowl. Pour the marinade over the smoked salmon. Cover everything with cling film and place in the fridge to marinate for 10 minutes. Cut the avocado in half-lengthwise, remove the outer skin and the central stone and then cut it into cubes. Wash the cucumber, cut it in half and with a mandolin, or a peeler if you do not have a mandolin, cut the cucumber into thin strips. Now take a bowl and put the salmon slices. You can also add the cucumber and diced avocado. Finish decorating the salad with sesame seeds; sprinkle everything with a little olive oil and a sprinkle of salt and pepper. You can serve the salad.

85.   Orange smoked salmon and mushrooms salad

PREPARATION TIME: 10 minutes + 30 minutes of rest in the fridge CALORIES: 215

INGREDIENTS FOR 2 SERVINGS

320 grams of smoked salmon 120 grams of mushrooms 30 ml of olive oil 1 orange 1 sprig of parsley Salt and pepper to taste.

DIRECTIONS

Squeeze the orange and take the juice. Remove the earthy part of the mushrooms, then wash, and dry them. Cut them into very thin slices. Put the mushrooms in a bowl, add salt, pepper, and half of the orange juice and mix everything very gently. Wash and dry the parsley and then chop it. Take two serving plates and place the salmon divided into equal parts on the bottom of the plate. Arrange the mushrooms on top of the salmon and then sprinkle with the chopped parsley. Take a small bowl and add the oil, the rest of the orange juice, a pinch of salt and pepper. With a fork, emulsify everything well. Sprinkle the mushrooms and salmon with the sauce and refrigerate to marinate for 20 minutes. Serve as soon as the marinade is finished in the fridge.

86.   Cod fillet and veggies

PREPARATION TIME: 15 minutes COOKING TIME: 12 minutes CALORIES: 290

INGREDIENTS FOR 2 SERVINGS

200 grams of clean cod fillet 100 grams of mushrooms 200 grams of green asparagus 1 teaspoon of chives 1 clove of garlic Olive oil Salt and pepper to taste

DIRECTIONS Start the recipe with cod. Wash the cod fillets, dry them with paper towel and remove skin and bones if still present. Sprinkle the fillets with a pinch of salt and a little pepper on both sides and set aside. Clean the mushrooms by removing the earthy part first. Wash them under running water, dry them and cut them into slices. Switch to the asparagus. Remove the hard stems, wash them under running water and then dry them. Peel the garlic and then wash it. Dry it and chop it finely. In a bowl, pour two tablespoons of oil, the minced garlic, the chives, a pinch of salt and the pepper. Stir and mix everything well. Take a baking pan and brush it with a drizzle of oil. Place the cod fillets on top and cover with the asparagus and mushrooms. Sprinkle everything with the marinade. In the meantime, you have preheated the oven to 180 ° C. cook the cod for at least 15 minutes. After 15 minutes check the cooking and if necessary, continue for another 5 minutes. Serve the cod with the vegetables.

87. Flavoured herbs cod

PREPARATION TIME: 15 minutes COOKING TIME: 15/20 minutes CALORIES: 390

INGREDIENTS FOR 2 SERVINGS

2 cod fillets of about 200 grams for each 1 teaspoon of rosemary 1 garlic clove 1 sage leaf 1 teaspoon of chopped parsley Salt and pepper to taste. 1 pinch of dried oregano 1 tablespoon of coconut oil

DIRECTIONS

First, rinse the cod under running water. After cleaning it, let it dry thoroughly. Add all the aromatic herbs and mix. Mix the herbs with a few drops of lemon and a little coconut oil. Let it soak for a few minutes. Once macerated, spread the marinade on both sides of the cod. Place the fish on a baking pan. Bake preheated oven for 15 min at 180 °C. Always check the cooking and if the fish is not ready, cook for another 5 minutes. When cooked, you can serve the cod flavoured with herbs.

88.   Hazelnut crusted cod

PREPARATION TIME: 15 minutes COOKING TIME: 5 minutes
CALORIES: 340

INGREDIENTS FOR 2 SERVINGS

2 cod fillets of 200 grams for each 50 grams of chopped
hazelnuts 1 teaspoon of soy yogurt 2 tablespoons of olive oil
Salt and Pepper to taste.

DIRECTIONS

Take the cod fillet, wash it and rinse it. Now dry it with a paper
towel. Cut it lengthwise to obtain slices. Try not to cut too thick
slices. Put the cod slices in a baking dish and sprinkle them
with a little olive oil and soy yogurt. Season them with, salt and
pepper. If you do not have chopped hazelnuts, you can take
them whole and chop them yourself. Take the slices of cod and
pass them in the peanut breading making sure to press well so
that it is breaded on all sides. Put a tablespoon of oil in a non-
stick pan and let it heat up. As soon as the oil starts to sizzle,
put the breaded fish slices in the pan and cook them for a couple
of minutes on both sides. Cook until cod is soft. As soon as the
cod is cooked, place it on a serving dish and serve.

89. Sea bass and cherry tomatoes

PREPARATION TIME: 15 minutes COOKING TIME: 20 minutes CALORIES: 361

INGREDIENTS FOR 2 SERVINGS

2 sea bass of 200 grams each (already cleaned) A garlic clove A small shallot 200 grams of cherry tomatoes 2 tablespoons of lime juice Oregano to taste Salt and pepper to taste. Olive oil to taste

DIRECTIONS

Wash the sea bass under running water. Let it drain for a few minutes and dry them with a paper towel. Peel the shallot, wash it and then chop it. Peel the garlic, wash it and then chop it. Take a baking dish, brush it with a little oil and then lay the fish on top. Drizzle with oil and sprinkle with the chopped garlic and shallot. Wash the cherry tomatoes, dry them and cut them in half. Spread the cherry tomatoes over the fish and sprinkle with salt, pepper and oregano. Put the dish in the oven preheated to 180 ° C for 15 minutes. After 5 minutes, take the sea bass out of the oven and sprinkle it with the lime juice and then cook for another 5 minutes., Check the cooking and if they do not seem cooked enough, continue cooking for another 2 minutes. Serve the sea bass with the cherry tomatoes still hot

90. Kiwi salad

PREPARATION TIME: 30 minutes COOKING TIME: 30 minutes CALORIES: 167

INGREDIENTS FOR 2 SERVINGS

2 kiwis 1 yellow pepper The juice of half a lemon 70 grams of cooked corn 50 grams of tofu 4 cherry tomatoes Olive oil to taste Salt and pepper to taste

DIRECTIONS

Peel the kiwis, wash them, cut them in two and then slice them. Wash the peppers then remove the seeds and internal filaments and cut them into slices. Wash the cherry tomatoes and then cut each of them into 4 wedges. Put tomatoes, kiwis and peppers in a salad bowl. Rinse and pat the tofu with absorbent paper and then put it to grill for two minutes on each side. Remove the tofu from the grill, cut it into cubes and put it in the salad bowl. Add the corn and mix. In a bowl put the lemon juice, salt, pepper and olive oil and mix with a fork. Sprinkle the vegetables and tofu with the emulsion. Mix well and serve.

91. Corn soup

PREPARATION TIME: 10 minutes COOKING TIME: 20 minutes CALORIES: 151

INGREDIENTS FOR 2 SERVINGS

200 grams of corn kernels Half a shallot 500 ml of vegetable broth Olive oil to taste Salt and pepper to taste

DIRECTIONS

Peel and wash the shallot and then chop it. Heat up a little oil in a saucepan and then put the shallot to brown for a couple of minutes. Add the corn kernels and mix. Sauté the corn for a couple of minutes and then add the vegetable broth. Cook for 20 minutes. Season with salt and pepper, mix and turn off. Take an immersion blender and coarsely blend the corn. Put the soup on serving plates, season with a drizzle of oil and serve.

92.   Potato soup with Saffron

PREPARATION TIME: 10 minutes COOKING TIME: 30 minutes CALORIES: 220

INGREDIENTS FOR 2 SERVINGS

3 small potatoes 1 small carrot 1 shallot 2 saffron tubs 700 ml of vegetable broth Chopped chives to taste Salt and pepper to taste Olive oil to taste

DIRECTIONS

Peel and wash the carrot and then cut it into pieces. Peel, wash and chop the shallot. Peel and wash the potatoes thoroughly and then cut them into cubes. Heat up a little oil in a saucepan and then brown the shallot. Add the carrot, potatoes, and mix. Let it cook for 5 minutes and then add the vegetable broth. Cook until the vegetables are tender. Season with salt and pepper and add the saffron sachets. Mix well and cook for another two minutes. Turn off and with an immersion blender blend everything until you get a creamy and velvety mixture. Put on serving plates, season with oil and pepper, decorate with chives and serve.

93. Brown rice with tomato

PREPARATION TIME: 15 minutes COOKING TIME: 40 minutes CALORIES: 321

INGREDIENTS FOR 2 SERVINGS

120 grams of brown rice 250 gr of tomato pulp Half a shallot 400 ml of vegetable broth 2 chopped basil leaves Salt and pepper to taste Olive oil to taste

DIRECTIONS

Peel the shallot and chop it. Put some oil in a saucepan and when it is hot, put the shallot and basil to fry. When the shallot is golden brown, add the tomato pulp. Mix, season with salt, pepper, and cook for 20 minutes. In the meantime, put the vegetable broth in a saucepan and bring to a boil. Now put the rice to cook for about twenty minutes. When it is cooked, drain it and put it in the pot with the tomato. Mix thoroughly and then put the rice on serving plates. Season with a drizzle of oil and serve.

94.　Turmeric potatoes

PREPARATION TIME: 15 minutes COOKING TIME: 40 minutes CALORIES: 214

INGREDIENTS FOR 2 SERVINGS

4 potatoes 1 teaspoon of turmeric powder 1 sprig of rosemary 1 clove of garlic Salt and pepper to taste Olive oil to taste

DIRECTIONS

Peel the potatoes, wash them carefully and cut them into regular chunks. Put the potatoes in a bowl. In a small bowl put oil, salt, pepper, turmeric, and mix until you get a homogeneous emulsion. Peel and wash the garlic and then cut it into slices. Put the garlic in the bowl with the potatoes. Season everything with the turmeric emulsion and mix well. Take a baking sheet and line it with baking paper. Pour the potatoes with all the contents of the bowl. Put in the oven and cook at 200 ° C for 40 minutes. As soon as they are cooked, take them out of the oven and serve them immediately.

95.   Sweet and sour fennel

PREPARATION TIME: 15 minutes COOKING TIME: 20 minutes CALORIES: 138

INGREDIENTS FOR 2 SERVINGS

2 small fennels 2 tablespoons of apple cider vinegar 2 teaspoons of toasted pine nuts 6 black olives 1 teaspoon of honey Olive oil to taste Salt and pepper to taste

DIRECTIONS

Remove the hard outer part of the fennel, then wash them and cut them into 8 wedges. Put them to boil for 5 minutes in boiling salted water. After 5 minutes turn off and let them drain. Heat a drizzle of olive oil in a pan and when it is hot put the fennel to sauté for a couple of minutes. Season with salt, pepper, and mix. Add the vinegar and honey and mix again. Now add the toasted pine nuts and cook for another 2 minutes. Turn off, put the fennel in serving dishes and serve.

96. Avocado and cucumber tartare

PREPARATION TIME: 20 minutes CALORIES: 230

INGREDIENTS FOR 2 SERVINGS

2 small cucumbers Half a lemon 1 small avocado Half a shallot
Olive oil to taste Salt and pepper to taste

DIRECTIONS

Remove the tips of the gherkins, then wash them and cut them
into cubes. Peel the avocado, cut it in half, remove the stone,
then wash it, and cut it into cubes. Put the avocado and
cucumber in a bowl. Peel and wash the shallot and then chop it
and place it in the bowl with the cucumber and avocado. Season
with lemon juice, oil, salt and pepper and mix well. Place a
pastry cutter in the centre of the serving dish. With a spoon
take the mixture and fill the inside of the pastry ring. Remove
the pastry rings and serve.

97.   Salad of cucumbers, radishes, rocket and olives

PREPARATION TIME: 20 minutes CALORIES: 120

INGREDIENTS FOR 2 SERVINGS

1 cucumber 4 radishes 50 grams of rocket 6 black olives a jar
of soy yogurt salt and pepper to taste olive oil to taste

DIRECTIONS

Wash the radishes carefully, remove the roots and then cut
them into rings. Wash and dry the rocket Wash the cucumber
and then cut it into slices. Put the vegetables in a salad bowl. In
a separate bowl put the yogurt, oil, salt, pepper and oregano.
With a fork mix everything well. Put the olives in the bowl with
the vegetables and mix. Season them with oil, salt and pepper
and then put them on serving plates. Sprinkle with the yogurt
sauce and serve.

98.   Orange seitan steaks

PREPARATION TIME: 10 minutes COOKING TIME: 20 minutes CALORIES: 157

INGREDIENTS FOR 2 SERVINGS

120 grams of seitan 1 orange Half a lemon Olive oil to taste Salt and pepper to taste

DIRECTIONS

Rinse and pat the seitan with absorbent paper, then cut it into slices. Put a little olive oil in a pan and as soon as it is hot, cook the slices of seitan, two minutes per side. Put the slices aside and in the same pan put the filtered orange and lemon juice. Bring to a boil, season with salt and pepper and mix. Now put the slices of seitan in the pan let them flavour for a couple of minutes and then turn off. Put the slices on serving plates, sprinkle with the cooking juices and serve.

99.   Grilled tofu and beetroot skewers

PREPARATION TIME: 25 minutes COOKING TIME: 25 minutes CALORIES: 177

INGREDIENTS FOR 2 SERVINGS

120 grams of tofu 4 mint leaves 120 grams of cooked beets a teaspoon of honey 1 orange 2 tablespoons of balsamic vinegar olive oil to taste salt and pepper to taste

DIRECTIONS

Rinse and then pat the tofu with absorbent paper. Cut it into cubes. Wash and dry the orange, grate the zest and strain the juice into a bowl. Wash and dry the mint leaves. Put the balsamic vinegar, orange juice, honey, orange zest and a little pepper in a saucepan. Bring to a boil, lower the heat and cook the sauce until it is thick. Peel the beets and cut them into 6 wedges. Emulsify the filtered lemon juice, oil, salt and pepper in a bowl. Now take the skewer sticks and put the beetroot cubes first, then the tofu cubes. Continue until the ingredients are finished. Now put a mint leaf on each skewer. Brush the skewers with the lemon oil emulsion. Reheat a grill and place the skewers to grill for two minutes per side. Place the skewers on serving plates, sprinkle with the balsamic vinegar sauce and serve.

100. Spicy grilled zucchini

PREPARATION TIME: 10 minutes COOKING TIME: 10 minutes CALORIES: 87

INGREDIENTS FOR 2 SERVINGS

2 zucchinis 1 clove of garlic 1 hot pepper Olive oil to taste Salt and pepper to taste

DIRECTIONS

Start by preparing the chili oil. Peel the garlic, wash it and then cut it in half. Wash and chop the chilli Put the garlic and chilli in a bowl and cover them with olive oil. Set aside until the zucchinis are cooked. Now remove the tips from the zucchinis, wash them and cut them into thin slices. Sprinkle them with salt and pepper and then put them to grill on a hot grill. When they are cooked, place in a serving dish, season with the chilli oil and serve.

101.   Zucchini, peppers and mushrooms in a pan

PREPARATION TIME: 10 minutes COOKING TIME: 20 minutes CALORIES: 93

INGREDIENTS FOR 2 SERVINGS

1 yellow pepper 1 zucchini 200 grams of mushrooms 4 chopped basil leaves Olive oil to taste Salt and pepper to taste

DIRECTIONS

Remove the tips from the zucchinis, wash them and cut them into thin cubes. Proceed with the pepper, wash it and remove the top cap. With a sharp knife, remove all seeds and internal filaments, cut the pepper into strips and divide them in half. Remove the earthy part of the mushrooms, wash them, dry them and then cut them into slices. In a large non-stick pan, heat a tablespoon of oil and pour the pepper inside first. Sauté them for a few minutes and add the courgettes to the pan. Stir occasionally for even cooking and cook over high heat adding about 1 glass of water. When the water is almost all absorbed, add the mushrooms. Season with salt and pepper and mix well. Cook until the vegetables are soft. At this point, turn off, season with chopped basil and serve.

102. Pumpkin in a pan with onions

PREPARATION TIME: 15 minutes COOKING TIME: 30 minutes CALORIES: 71

INGREDIENTS FOR 2 SERVINGS

200 grams of pumpkin pulp 1 red onion 200 ml of vegetable broth Salt and pepper to taste Olive oil to taste

DIRECTIONS

Wash the pumpkin pulp and then cut it into cubes. Peel and wash the onion and then cut it into slices. Heat some oil in a pan and as soon as it is hot, brown the onion for a couple of minutes. Add the pumpkin, season with salt and pepper and mix. Cook the pumpkin for a couple of minutes and then add the broth. Cover the pan with a lid and cook for 30 minutes. After 30 minutes, turn off, season the pumpkin with a little oil and pepper and serve.

103. Green beans, potatoes and zucchini

PREPARATION TIME: 20 minutes COOKING TIME: 40 minutes CALORIES: 285

INGREDIENTS FOR 2 SERVINGS

100 grams of green beans 1 potato 10 cherry tomatoes 1 zucchini Olive oil to taste Salt and pepper to taste

DIRECTIONS

Wash the potato with all the peel and then cook it for 20 minutes in boiling salted water. Remove the tips from the green beans, wash them and then cook them in boiling salted water for 15 minutes. Wash the cherry tomatoes and then cut them in half. Wash the zucchini and then cut it into cubes. Drain the potato, pass it under cold water and then peel it and cut it into cubes. Drain the green beans and then cut them in half. In a pan, heat a tablespoon of olive oil and as soon as it is hot, add the zucchini. Cook for 5 minutes, and then add the cherry tomatoes. Stir, let it salt for 2 minutes and then add the green beans and the potato. Cook for 2-3 minutes. Season with salt and pepper, stir and then turn off. Put on plates and serve.

104. Peppers and green beans

PREPARATION TIME: 30 minutes COOKING TIME: 20 minutes CALORIES: 160

INGREDIENTS FOR 2 SERVINGS

1 yellow pepper 1 red pepper 150 grams of green beans 2 tomatoes half a shallot olive oil to taste salt and pepper to taste

DIRECTIONS

Peel and wash the shallot and then chop it. Cut the peppers in half, remove the seeds and white filaments, then wash them and cut them into cubes. Wash the tomatoes and cut them into cubes. Remove the tips from the green beans, wash them and then cook them in boiling salted water for 15 minutes. As soon as they are cooked, drain and let them cool and then cut them into small pieces. Fry the shallot in a pan with a tablespoon of oil. Add the tomatoes and cubes, stir and sauté for a couple of minutes. Now add the peppers and green beans. Season with salt, pepper, and mix. Add a glass of water and cook with the lid on until all the vegetables are soft. As soon as they are cooked, turn off, put on plates and serve.

105. Brown rice with vegetables and olives

PREPARATION TIME: 25 minutes COOKING TIME: 35 minutes CALORIES: 405

INGREDIENTS FOR 2 SERVINGS

140 grams of brown rice 1 zucchini 1 small eggplant 6 black olives 4 cherry tomatoes 500 ml of vegetable broth Olive oil to taste Salt and pepper to taste

DIRECTIONS

Wash the zucchini and eggplant and then cut it into cubes. Wash the cherry tomatoes and cut them in half. Cut the olives in half and remove the stone. Brush a baking sheet with olive oil and then put the vegetables inside. Season with oil, salt, pepper, and mix. Put them in the oven and cook at 200 ° c for 35 minutes. In the meantime, prepare the rice. Put the vegetable broth in a saucepan and bring to a boil. Now add the rice and cook for 20 minutes. As soon as it is cooked, drain it and put it in a bowl. Take the vegetables out of the oven and then put them in the bowl with the rice. Season with oil, salt and pepper, mix and serve.

106. Seitan with mango

PREPARATION TIME: 20 minutes+ 60 minutes to rest in fridge COOKING TIME: 15 minutes CALORIES: 267

INGREDIENTS FOR 2 SERVINGS

200 grams of seitan 1 mango 1 tablespoon of soy sauce A teaspoon of honey Salt and pepper to taste Olive oil to taste Sesame seeds to taste

DIRECTIONS

Peel and wash the mango and then cut it into pieces. Put it in a bowl and press it with a fork. Now add the soy sauce, honey, a tablespoon of olive oil, salt and pepper. Mix everything well. Dab the seitan with absorbent paper and then cut it into slices. Put the seitan in the bowl with the mango. Cover the bowl with transparent paper and put in the fridge to marinate for an hour. After the marinating time, take a baking sheet and brush it with olive oil. Pour all the contents of the bowl into the baking sheet and put in the oven. Cook for 15 minutes at 200 ° C. As soon as it is cooked, remove from the oven, put the seitan and the side dish on serving plates and serve.

107. Potato and caper salad

PREPARATION TIME: 15 minutes COOKING TIME: 30 minutes CALORIES: 200

INGREDIENTS FOR 2 SERVINGS

400 grams of potatoes A teaspoon of capers A sprig of chopped parsley Two chopped basil leaves Olive oil to taste Apple cider vinegar to taste Salt and pepper to taste

DIRECTIONS

Wash the potatoes without peeling them, and then cook them for 30 minutes in plenty of salted water. Drain and let them cool. Once warm, peel the potatoes and place them on a cutting board. Now cut the potatoes into not too small cubes. Put the potatoes in a salad bowl. Rinse the capers, pat them with absorbent paper and then chop them. Put them in a bowl with the basil, parsley and vinegar. Add salt, pepper and a tablespoon of olive oil and mix well with a fork. Pour the emulsion over the potatoes and mix to flavour well. Now you can serve.